The Healthcare IT Environment

Strategies for Providers and Vendors

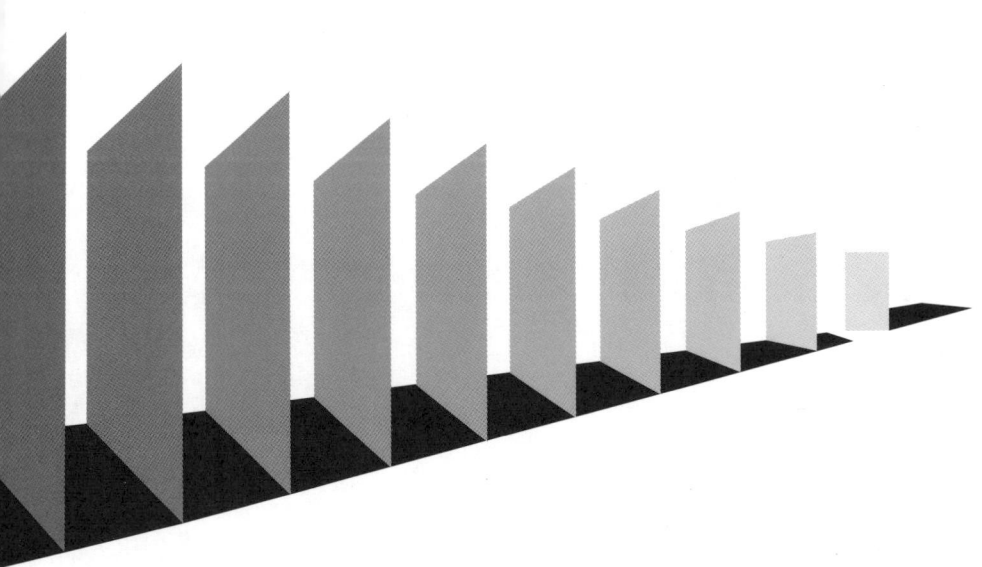

SPONSORED BY

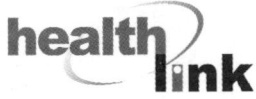

HEALTHCARE INFORMATION AND MANAGEMENT SYSTEMS SOCIETY

Copyright ©*2001*

Healthcare Information and Management Systems Society
230 E. Ohio St.
Suite 500
Chicago, IL 60611

All rights reserved. This book is protected by copyright. No part of this book may be reproduced in any form or by any means, including photocopying, or utilized by any information storage and retrieval system without written permission from the copyright owner.

ISBN 0-9715301-3-0

Table of Contents

Introduction 1

Section 1.0 – Societal/Cultural/Demographic Trends 3
1.1 Changing Demographics 3
1.2 Rise of Consumerism/Use of Internet 8
1.3 Complementary and Alternative Medicine 13

Section 2.0 – Technology/E-Strategy 17
2.1 Electronic Medical Records/Clinical Information Systems 17
2.2 Changing Role of the Chief Information Officer 21
2.3 E-business Capabilities 23
2.4 Telemedicine/health 25

Section 3.0 – Scientific/Clinical Trends 31
3.1 Advances in Genomics and Biotechnology 31
3.2 Improving Quality of Care and Patient Safety 35

Section 4.0 – Government/Regulation 41
4.1 HIPAA/Privacy/Security Regulations 41
4.2 Regulation of Drug Costs 43

Section 5.0 – Economic/Reimbursement Trends 47
5.1 Healthcare Costs Increase 47
5.2 Financial Instability of Healthcare Organizations 49
5.3 Emergence of New Financing Models 53
5.4 Competition for Capital 56
5.5 Costs of Healthcare Shift to Consumer 58
5.6 Integration/Consolidation 59

Section 6.0 – Health Policy 65
6.1 Medicare and Medicaid Reform 65
6.2 The Uninsured 66

Section 7.0 – Human Capital 69
7.1 Human Resource Shortages 69
7.2 Unionization 71

Introduction

In the nineteenth century, a handful of critical scientific advances – ranging from aseptic surgery to anesthesia – helped to transform the art of healing from a crude trade applied by barber surgeons to an emerging scientific discipline. New advancements brought with them the hope of improved outcomes and, in the process, raised the cultural esteem and authority of the healing arts professions.

Though profound, these scientific and technical developments were not the sole source of change within healthcare. Rather, they were accompanied by a myriad of other environmental factors that aided in the transformation. Perhaps most critical were changes to medical education accompanied by strict new licensure requirements.

For the next hundred years, healthcare would continue to evolve at an astounding pace. Each decade would bring new knowledge, new technology and the further conquest of disease. The passage of time would also spawn new challenges, however. Chief among these has been the cost of care, which has continued to rise, seemingly inexorably, to now-dizzying heights.

Today, at the beginning of the twenty-first century, healthcare once again stands on the brink of a major transformation – one no less profound than that of the nineteenth century. Scientific, technological, legislative, economic, demographic and sociological factors are combining to reshape the face of what we call "healthcare." Undoubtedly, a century from now, historians will view this period as the dawning of a new era – one in which the promise of scientifically based healthcare was finally realized. Yet they will also examine how effectively society resolved the enormous ethical, economic and legal questions this change produced.

Admittedly, it is far easier to retrospectively analyze such times than live through them. The phenomenal pace of change today makes it difficult for healthcare-related organizations to develop and execute market-driven strategies in a timely fashion. Nonetheless, that is the challenge facing the numerous organizations that constitute the healthcare industry - including the information technology companies whose infrastructure will help form the foundation for much of the transformation to come.

Healthcare information and management systems professionals must understand the key factors that are transforming the healthcare landscape and their probable impact on the various components of the delivery system. The following environmental assessment identifies key drivers and expounds on the probable impact these emerging forces will have.

The purpose of this study is threefold:
- To provide healthcare information and management systems professionals with an analysis of key, current and forecasted environmental trends within the healthcare industry and to present an evolving picture of the healthcare landscape.

- To assess how these trends may impact the adoption of health information technology and thus create either opportunities or threats for vendors of health information systems.
- To provide templates or tools to aid these healthcare professionals in analyzing the maturation of these trends within their markets.

To identify the major trends in healthcare, a meta-analysis was conducted of existing environmental assessments. Documents from government agencies, healthcare professional and trade associations, consulting firms, healthcare and business journals, pharmaceutical companies, healthcare providers and the investment community provided the majority of the subject matter from which the trends were selected. These trends were collectively reviewed, prioritized, and narrowed to a list of 20 key trends across seven different categories. Additional research further illuminated each trend and provided a confidence level regarding the impact the trend is likely to have on the industry.

Based upon this research, a working draft was developed for circulation to individuals with extensive knowledge and experience in the areas addressed. This final document represents not only a synthesis of information from existing environmental assessments and subject matter experts, but it also introduces some novel thoughts on how healthcare organizations and technology companies can prepare for future changes and, at the same time, strengthen their positions in the marketplace.

A footnote: The aftermath of the horrific terrorist attacks on the World Trade Center and Pentagon on Sept. 11, 2001 is certain to provide new challenges for healthcare information and management systems professionals as the healthcare industry rushes to strengthen its security and emergency response initiatives. Many hospitals have already begun to upgrade their electronic surveillance and high-tech security monitoring systems, and introduce new procedures for screening visitors. Additionally, the healthcare industry is prioritizing efforts to seek long-term solutions to combating computer terrorism and improving the security of wireless devices in hospitals. All these efforts, however, will be incumbent on the short- and long-term effects the terrorist attacks could have on IT capital spending.

Section 1.0 – Societal/Cultural/Demographic Trends

1.1 Changing Demographics

Background

One of the most significant environmental factors likely to shape healthcare in the coming decades is the dramatic shift taking place within the population of the United States. In the years ahead, substantive changes will occur with respect to the average age, ethnicity, life expectancy, income and education of U.S. residents. Although these changes will impact all aspects of society, they will have a particularly strong effect on the healthcare environment.

Larger Elderly Population

The number of elderly in the United States will soon grow significantly due to two factors: (1) Aging baby boomers (individuals born between 1946 and 1964), and (2) continuing increases in life expectancy. Currently, 34.5 million U.S. citizens are over the age of 65 years. In 2010, when the first generation of baby boomers turns 65 years old, that number will increase to almost 45 million, a gain of approximately 30 percent. By 2030, individuals over the age of 65 years will make up 20 percent of the total population.

Since the turn of the century, life expectancies have steadily increased from 47 years of age for the average male up to the present level of almost 74 years (NCHS, Health, United States, 1999) (See Figure 1).

By 2010, it is projected that men will live on average to age 76 years and women to age 86 years (Institute for the Future, 2000). Much of this change can be attributed to improvements in public health, medicine and technology. Because people are living longer, the number of the "oldest old," or those over 85 years, will grow to 7 million in 2020 and double to 14 million by 2040 (See Figure 2).

Figure 1. Life Expectancy
Source: Life Expectancy 1937-97, National Center for Health Statistics, 7525 Belcrest Rd., Hyattsville, MD 22782, www.cdc.gov/nchs

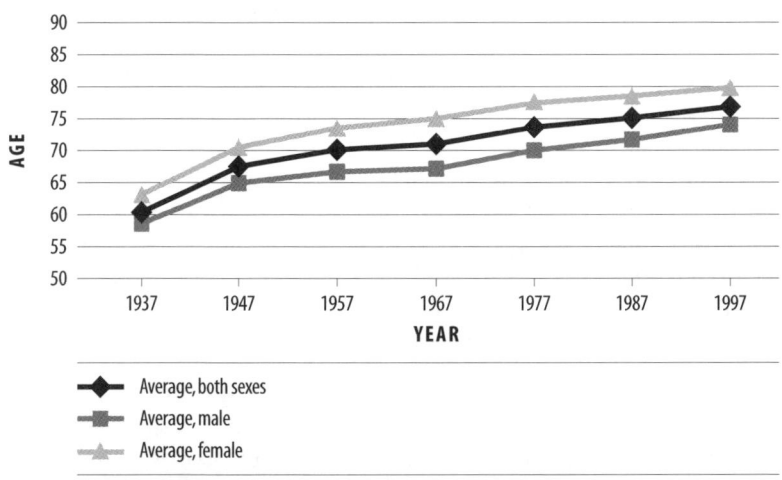

Figure 2. Total Number of Persons Age 65 or Older, By Age Group, 1900 to 2050, in millions
Source: Older Americans 2000: Key indicators of well-being, Federal Interagency on Aging Related Statistics

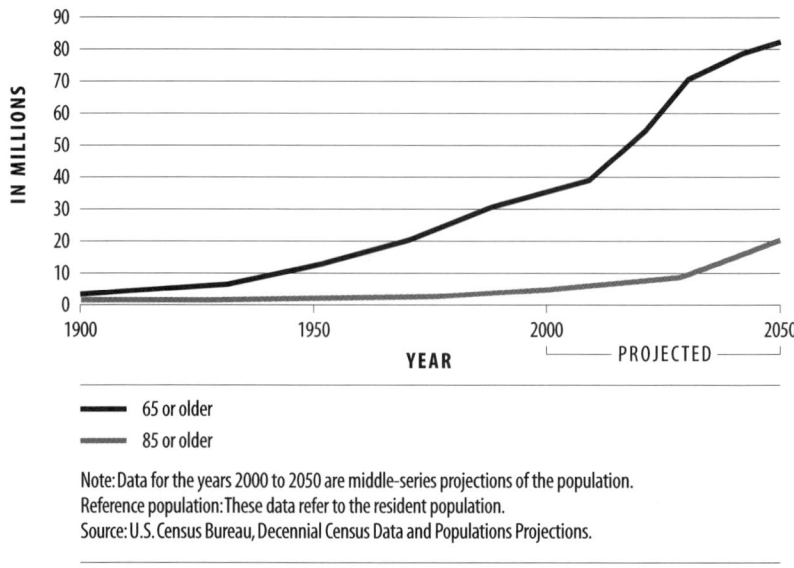

Note: Data for the years 2000 to 2050 are middle-series projections of the population.
Reference population: These data refer to the resident population.
Source: U.S. Census Bureau, Decennial Census Data and Populations Projections.

As individuals age, their need for healthcare services clearly increases. Indeed, the frequency, type and intensity of services required changes dramatically with age. Data from the 1998 National Health Interview Survey indicates that a population aged 45 to 64 years will likely utilize 678 days of care per 1,000 population, whereas those aged 65 years and over will utilize 1,496 days per 1,000 population. The elderly population's need for increased inpatient services typically reflects the complexity of their medical conditions, which is often accentuated by their relative fragility. Such patients many times are admitted with a primary diagnosis, yet possess multiple co-morbid conditions. This results in the need for a team of specialists within a healthcare facility to help deliver their care.

Ironically, the increasing forecast demand for healthcare services, including inpatient care, directly conflicts with the shift from inpatient to outpatient care that has occurred in the last decade (See Figure 3). In 1975, there were 687 hospital beds per 100,000 population. By 1998, that number had dropped to 378 beds (Henry J. Kaiser Family Foundation, *The Kaiser Changing Health Care Marketplace Project*, 1998). This decrease in staffed beds has been driven by several factors, including the presence of relatively stable admission rates for inpatient care accompanied by shorter lengths of stay. The average length of stay decreased from 6.0 days per admission in 1991 to 4.5 days by 1998 (Healthcare 2000, p. 58) (See Figure 4). In contrast, the number of outpatient encounters per 1,000 covered lives rose from 11,239 in 1991 to 17,184 in 1998. (See Figure 4) The convenience and lower cost of outpatient settings make them attractive to patients as well as to healthcare payers.

Although the elderly population is using more healthcare services in comparison to a younger population, they are still active and mobile and continue to serve as productive members of society. The percentage of Medicare beneficiaries who are chronically

Figure 3. Hospital Admissions and Outpatient Visits for the Past 10 Years
Source: Hospital Statistics, American Hospital Association, One North Franklin Street, Chicago IL. 60606, www.aha.org

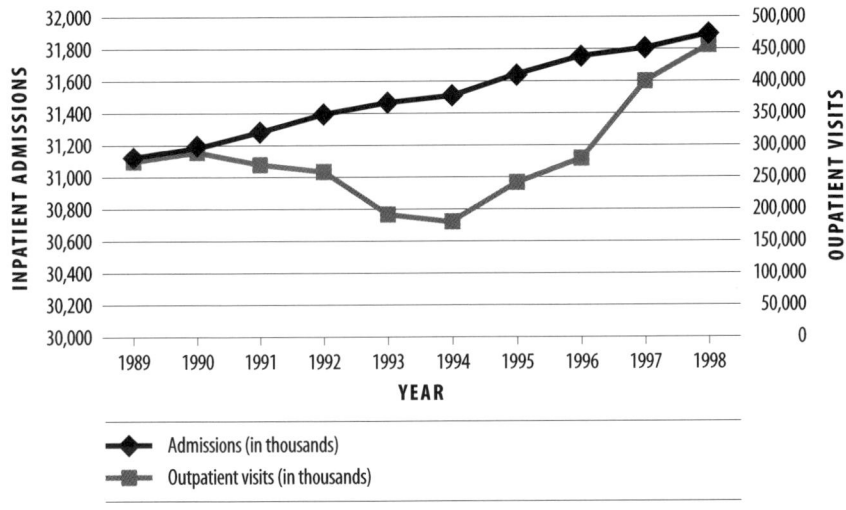

Figure 4. Average Length of Stay Continues to Decline
Source: The MEDSTAT Group MarketScan Database, 1999.

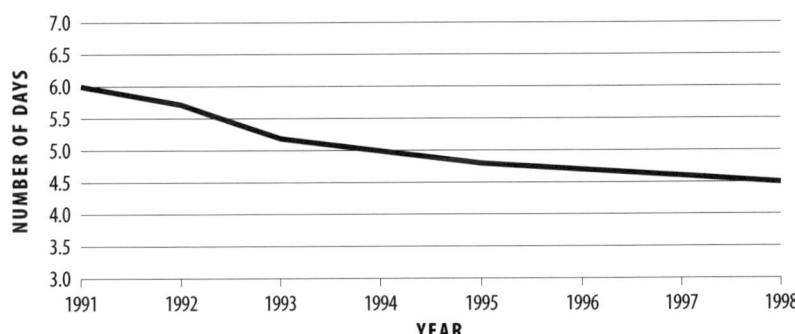

disabled has continually declined since 1984, and the percentage of elderly who report having a sedentary lifestyle is also decreasing. Even when no longer working, the elderly continue to engage in social and community activities. In 1995, more than 50 percent of those aged 70 years and older reported that they still go out to restaurants, 40 percent indicated they still attend church, and more than 80 percent maintain contact with friends or neighbors (Older Americans 2000: Key indicators of well-being, Federal Interagency on Aging Related Statistics).

Increasing Diversity
The ethnic roots of the United States will continue to become more diverse. Recent data indicates that 74 percent of the population is Caucasian. In the future, minority populations will account for a growing percentage of the total population, led by growth in the number of individuals with Asian/Pacific Islander and Hispanic origins.

Figure 5. Racial and Ethnic Distribution of the U.S. Population
Source: Bureau of Census, Statistical Abstract of the US, 1997 mid-projection series.

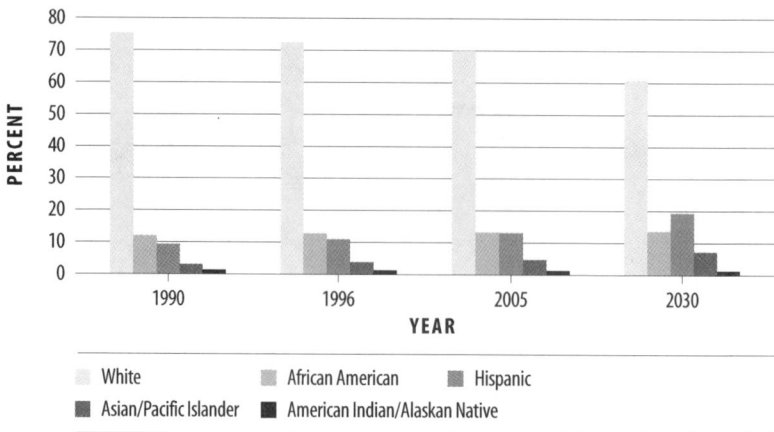

By 2010, the ethnic composition of the United States will be approximately 64 percent Caucasian, 13 percent African-American, 15 percent Hispanic, 5 percent Asian and less than one percent Native American (Institute for the Future, 2000) (See Figure 5).

The disparity in health status between members of different ethnic populations is notable. For example, infant mortality rates are 2.5 times higher for African-Americans and 1.5 times higher for American Indians than for whites. The rate of prostate cancer in African-American men is twice as high as the rate in white males. Diabetes is seen twice as much in Hispanics as in whites, and the prevalence of this disease in African-Americans is 70 percent higher than in the white population. Additionally, Hispanics at any level of family income are more likely to be uninsured than white or African-American families.

Although the current healthcare system does a poor job of addressing these ethnic differences, as our nation grows more ethnically diverse, the system will be forced to offer solutions to the health issues of these groups. Members of ethnic groups will seek healthcare providers who are aware of and sensitive to their language, cultural and religious differences. In fact, African-American physicians are five times more likely to treat African-American patients and Hispanic doctors are 2.5 times more likely to treat Hispanic patients than other physicians. At the same time, racial and ethnic minority adults are presently less likely than white adults to be satisfied with the quality of healthcare they receive (Health Care Rx: Access for All).

Improvements in Education, Income and Health Status
Positive correlations can be found among the economic, educational and health statuses of individuals. As the education and/or wealth of the elderly population improves, so should the health status. In 1999, according to the U.S. Census Bureau, only 70 percent of non-institutionalized elderly had completed high school. In comparison, 81 percent of individuals aged 55 to 64 had received a high school education.

Thus, as the population ages, more of the elderly will have benefited from a high school education. Additionally, median income levels for the elderly have been on the rise since the late 1950s. Knowing this makes it possible to infer that the health of the elderly population will continue to improve.

However, it is important to remember that this general trend is not seen in some subgroups of the elderly population. For example, in 1992, the average income of elderly white males was $15,276, versus $5,968 for Hispanic women. And, as mentioned previously, differences between the health statuses of different subpopulations are obvious. Still, the stereotype of the elderly being uneducated and on a tight fixed income will begin to weaken. The elderly will become more engaged in decision-making related to all aspects of their life, especially their healthcare. They will also have higher expectations and demands and have some disposable income to support choices.

Strategic Implications for Healthcare Organizations
1. Healthcare organizations should determine how to meet the increasing demand for more services. While healthcare providers are now "leaner" organizationally, they may need to rebuild their inpatient capacity to previous levels should the growing elderly population truly demand more services. This assertion is supported by 1999 data from the American Hospital Association showing that inpatient admissions rose for the first time in more than a decade by 1.75 percent.

2. The increased need for services will also create the necessity for additional staff to provide these services. The supply of physicians in metropolitan areas is usually considered adequate, although the balance between different specialties may not be distributed optimally. In contrast, the supply of nurses is inadequate and the situation continues to worsen (see Section 7.1 on Human Resources Shortages for more information). Healthcare providers must create efficiencies in the care delivery process so they are able to do "more with less."

3. Organizations should prepare to meet the demands of a more educated, more mobile, wealthier and healthier elderly population. Not only is the aging population increasingly better educated, mobile and affluent, but it is also more demanding. A new era of consumerism is emerging within healthcare whereby the voice of the market will finally overshadow the voice of providers.

4. Increasingly, healthcare providers will need to create programs and services that address cultural differences in healthcare needs and statuses. The ability to recognize that one size does not fit all when developing, implementing and marketing programs and services will contribute to an organization's success. Should healthcare providers hope to serve ethnic populations, they must understand their needs and address them specifically. For example, facilities must tailor services such as dietary and pastoral care to culturally diverse patients, have translators available and educate staff on cultural differences. Once these changes have been made, the provider must market these offerings in a culturally sensitive manner.

Strategic Implications for Health Information Technology Organizations
1. Because an elderly yet mobile population will seek healthcare in a multitude of settings, healthcare information technology (HIT) systems will be required to track information across a variety of settings and geographic locations. Although the elderly population's need for inpatient services may be high, increased inpatient utilization will, over time, decline somewhat as a result of scientific advancements that allow for better management of chronic conditions in lower acuity settings. This diversity of healthcare delivery venues makes it imperative that HIT systems possess the ability to aggregate patient information, in real time, from a broad array of clinical settings.

2. HIT systems must create efficiencies in the care delivery process to allow healthcare providers to do "more with less." For example, efficiencies realized through such technologies as automated voice documentation and computerized physician order entry (CPOE) systems will help alleviate some of the time constraint issues inherent to the current nursing shortage. Additionally, increased demand on the healthcare system, coupled with the possibility of increased restrictive reimbursement, will force hospitals to transform their provision of care. Maximization of efficiency and efficacy through minimization of variation in clinical processes will reshape healthcare from a cottage industry into smoothly operating "factories" of care capable of meeting the complete healthcare needs of the population in an effective fashion.

3. Increased opportunities for disease management systems will present themselves as the elderly population segment grows in magnitude. Disease management systems could prove instrumental in ensuring that the care delivered to those afflicted with chronic disease is efficient and effective. This approach also could lower the frequency of high-acuity episodes for disease conditions such as diabetes, congestive heart failure and asthma.

Barriers
1. The financial constraints faced by healthcare providers make it difficult to build more facilities and invest in IT resources.
2. The improved health of the elderly may make the demand for healthcare services less than current trends would indicate.

1.2 Rise of Consumerism/Use of Internet

Background
According to Webster's dictionary, consumerism is the "promotion of the consumer's interests." From a healthcare perspective, it is a term used to refer to an attitudinal shift amongst a large section of the population whereby passive acceptance of healthcare services has been replaced by a more activist approach. The rise of consumerism in healthcare essentially means that patients have become more active participants in their care. Gone are the days when most patients would follow the recommendations of their physicians without question. Consumers are obtaining more information

about the effectiveness of their care and their providers, and they prefer to have a voice in decision-making. They also expect greater choice, respect, convenience and control; not unlike what they've come to expect from retailers or other service industries. Attempts to pass a Patients' Bill of Rights are but one example of how consumers are aggressively seeking to protect their right to be involved in their healthcare and to hold healthcare providers and insurers accountable for their actions.

Consumerism has led to an increased customer service orientation within many healthcare organizations. Providers are adopting service excellence strategies in hopes of not only improving patient satisfaction, but also enhancing financial performance and clinical outcomes. It is now common for mission statements to reflect a commitment to service and strategic plans to include initiatives aimed at furthering customer satisfaction. It is clear that those facilities that do not respond to this new orientation risk losing patients to the competition. A recent study by J.E. Ware showed that patients who rate their experience in a healthcare facility as "excellent" would recommend that provider to a friend 80 to 90 percent of the time, whereas someone who rated it as "good" would only make the recommendation 10 percent of the time (Health Care Strategic Management, *Can we afford a customer service initiative?* April 2000). As a result, the costs of not implementing customer service initiatives can be very high.

Many factors are driving the rise in consumerism. As mentioned previously, changing demographics, namely higher levels of income and education, have largely contributed to increasing consumer empowerment. Individuals now seek and understand more medical information and search for the best care. Many also have the luxury of using their disposable income to travel to distant locations to access healthcare services if dissatisfied with local offerings.

A second factor in the rise of consumerism is the Internet. The Internet provides consumers with a wealth of information in a way that is timely, inexpensive and accessible. In 1997, 43 percent of adults used the Internet to obtain health information (Future of the Internet in Health Care, 1999). Searches for health-related content alternated with pornography as the number-one search topic for the Web. Baby boomers make up one of the largest groups of online health information users. Popular health-related topics of interest include disease-related information, diet and nutrition, pharmaceuticals, women's health and fitness (Health Care 2000, p. 121). Unfortunately, the quality and reliability of online healthcare content varies widely. In a study of the quality of medical information found on the Internet, more than 99 percent of the information sources did not disclose conflicts of interest and more than 80 percent did not provide the credentials of the author or the date the information was posted (See Figure 6).

Despite these limitations, the use of the Internet for health information will continue to increase. By 2005, it is estimated that more than half of U.S. consumers will have access to a computer (Future of Internet and Health, 1999) and 88.5 million adults will use the Internet to find health information, shop for health products, and communicate with affiliated payers and providers (www.cyberdialogue.com) (See Figure 7).

Figure 6. Poor Quality of Medical Information on the Web – Attributes of 629 Pages Retrieved in 50 Searches to Answer Common Clinical Questions
Source: Hersh W, Gorman P, Sachered L. "Applicability and Quality of Information for Answering Clinical Questions on the Web." JAMA 1998; 280: 1307-08.

Don't disclose conflicts of interest	99%
Not applicable to the question that prompted the search	89%
Don't give date posted or updated	82%
Don't give authors' credentials	80%
Don't indicate author	69%
Not oriented to health care professionals	60%
Evidence-based resources	1%

Figure 7. Forecast of e-Health Consumers
Source: Cyber Dialogue, www.cyberdialogue.com

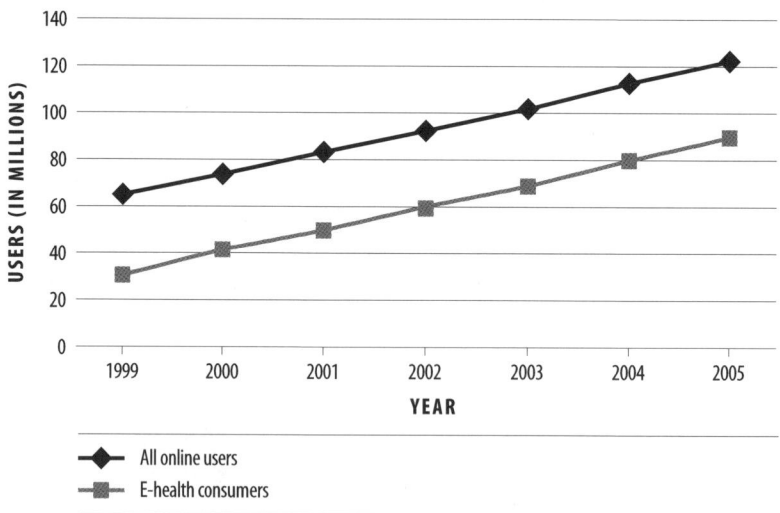

Research conducted by the Leifer Group indicates that physicians are already feeling the impact of consumerism, and specifically the use of the Internet, in their daily practice. Patients often independently research treatment options and present information gathered from the Internet for their doctor to review. Unfortunately, much of this information is not pertinent to the patient's specific case. In addition, the amount of time required to cull through this information with the patient not only is time taken away from the provision of care, but also imposes a time burden on physicians already struggling to optimize their efficiency as a result of decreased reimbursements from managed care organizations.

In a 1999 survey by PricewaterhouseCoopers, only 25 percent of healthcare executives surveyed agreed or strongly agreed that hospitals were prepared to handle the demands of an empowered customer (Healthcast 2010, 1999). To prepare, healthcare entities may need to realign organizational priorities, as well as reimbursement methods, to meet consumers' expanding expectations of customer service and clinical care that produces optimal outcomes.

Strategic Implications for Healthcare Organizations

1. Although the majority of healthcare providers have websites in place, most are first-generation "brochure-ware" used primarily for marketing, employee recruitment, online provider directories, and limited consumer health information (HIMSS Leadership Survey, 2000). Few websites have matured to the second generation whereby customized content and moderate interactivity occur. The next level of website development will involve transactions and the delivery of online care support. Very few providers have advanced to this state. Determining what healthcare consumers are looking for on an organization's website could be the first step in determining the best strategy for website enhancement.

2. Rather than being an enabler for the physician, the Internet, in the short-term, is proving to be a "disabler" because of the additional burden imposed on physicians by patients clamoring to have their latest search results validated. New tools are needed to enhance the consumer's ability to obtain precise, concise and valid data on medical conditions – information that holds up to intense physician scrutiny. Physicians must also determine how they will respond to patient e-mails in a manner that improves patient satisfaction through enhanced access, while not degrading the efficiency of the physicians' practices.

3. Create a culture of service excellence that recognizes that the "high-touch" attributes of care are as important to the consumer as clinical attributes of care. Because the vast majority of consumers are unable to differentiate between providers based upon clinical metrics, they often determine quality predicated on a subjective assessment of high-touch attributes. These attributes can include ease of access, waiting times for examinations or procedures, quality of food service, staff responsiveness to patient requests, and ambience and environment. Most hospitals measure patient satisfaction across these variables – looking for longitudinal trends, as well as comparisons to benchmark performance.

   When deficiencies are spotted, provider organizations generally make some effort to improve satisfaction with that particular measure. Though laudable, the path toward true service excellence requires far more than reacting to negative information gleaned from surveys. It requires a profound commitment to transform the organizational culture in a way that recognizes that a provider exists to meet the needs of its patients. A truly patient-centered culture requires not only significant engineering or reengineering of select processes, but the requisite technology to support and then automate these new processes.

4. Employee training and attitudes. Create advocates, intermediaries or service center that can help consumers navigate the system more effectively. The most precisely engineered systems will fail to deliver the expected value in terms of service excellence unless the staff is appropriately trained. Such training requires a significant amount of resources and also pulls workers from the provision of care at a time when most healthcare organizations are significantly understaffed.

5. Devote resources to branding and building customer loyalty. Healthcare entities could learn from the example of the pharmaceutical companies in marketing directly to the consumer and developing brand identity. Branding can be a powerful tool to clearly communicate an organization's strengths. The Internet will expand competitive boundaries. Competitors will not just be other healthcare organizations in a given geographic area, but they will include facilities throughout the nation that are targeting potential customers via the Internet. Consumers who in the past may not have known much about facilities throughout the nation will have ready access to this information. Already, MD Anderson Cancer Center in Houston, Texas, draws more than 75 percent of patients from outside its local service area. The organization has established a website that provides comprehensive information about the depth, breadth and quality of care provided and also allows patients to self-refer via the Internet.

6. Provide secure platform for the electronic exchange of information. Far from being an option, the provision of secure platforms is mandated by HIPAA and will become increasingly important as the use of ubiquitous electronic medical records becomes the norm. Patients will quickly lose faith in providers that are unable to ensure the privacy and sanctity of medical records, whether in electronic or paper form.

7. Involve consumers in decision-making. By definition, a patient-centered organization will include the patient when making important decisions. It also will frequently solicit the consumer's opinions on key issues by using a variety of venues, from focus groups to community boards.

Strategic Implications for Health Information Technology Organizations

1. The HIT industry must accelerate the development and deployment of e-health solutions that enhance the consumers' ability to access information, products and care delivery. The industry must also take a leadership role in identifying how, when and where personal health information will reside, as well as how it will be protected.

2. Vendors must demonstrate how HIT will contribute to providers' differentiation and competitive advantage. Just as consumers fail to differentiate between healthcare providers based upon clinical quality, it seems improbable that consumers will make selections based upon the presence or absence of HIT. Conversely, most consumers will be able to differentiate between providers based upon the benefits delivered by the provider's underlying health information technology. Thus, a hospital or ambulatory delivery site might promote its superb patient safety record, although it would probably not address the technological changes that have facilitated this accomplishment.

3. Vendors must directly market their products as a key component of high-quality care delivery, establishing brand-name recognition with consumers. In a tightly managed marketplace, little opportunity exists for the consumer to exercise his or her will when selecting providers. Hence, consumer marketing, other than for out-of-pocket or elective procedures, seems a bit oxymoronic. However, as steerage

becomes less of an issue, and the informed consumer is increasingly empowered to select his or her providers, direct marketing will emerge as an essential function for HIT vendors.

4. Customer relations management (CRM) systems should be adapted to healthcare. The value of CRM systems and principles has been well demonstrated in other industries. It's now healthcare's turn to evaluate the applicability of such applications within a variety of settings.

1.3 Complementary and Alternative Medicine

Background

A 1997 article in the *Journal of the American Medical Association* reported that 42 percent of Americans used some form of complementary medicine (Eisenberg et al, 1998). The study also suggested that the number of visits to alternative medicine providers exceeded those to primary care physicians. Complementary and alternative medicine (CAM) has grown into a $45 million industry and is expected to continue to grow 10 to 15 percent annually (Hospitals and Health Networks, November 2000). If spending for vitamins and herbs is included in these figures, CAM becomes a multi-billion dollar industry.

CAM includes a broad range of practices and philosophies, such as homeopathy, acupuncture, herbal therapies, massage therapy and chiropractic services. Despite the fact that many "traditional" healthcare providers believe that CAM does not have a role within Western medicine, other providers have now incorporated complementary medicine modalities into their daily practice. The change in healthcare providers' attitudes and beliefs has been driven not only by consumer demand, but also by scientific research.

In 1998, the government established the National Center for Complementary and Alternative Medicine (NCCAM) as part of the National Institutes of Health (NIH). The NCCAM develops and supports research to provide scientific evidence that different forms of complementary medicine can contribute to positive clinical outcomes and improved quality of life. The center also serves as a clearinghouse for information on alternative therapies. In addition, 75 out of 117 U.S. medical schools now offer an elective course in CAM. Consequently, the role of complementary medicine is slowly being integrated into the foundations upon which the best clinical care is based.

Consumers who use complementary medicine generally have higher levels of education and poorer overall health than the average population. They tend to use the non-traditional therapies as complements to traditional medicine, as opposed to alternatives. Proponents of CAM have high expectations for how quickly the integration of Eastern and Western medical practices can occur and who should pay for non-traditional approaches to care. Consumers believe health plans should pay for such services, but if not, it is likely that many consumers will continue to pay for CAM services out of pocket (Eisenberg et al, 1998). Less than 50 percent of spending for CAM currently is covered by insurance. Chiropractic services are the most common type of CAM to be covered. Some states, however, are considering legislation related to the licensing,

Figure 8. Alternative Therapies by Region
Source: US Hospitals and the Future of Health Care, Eighth Edition 2000, page 33.

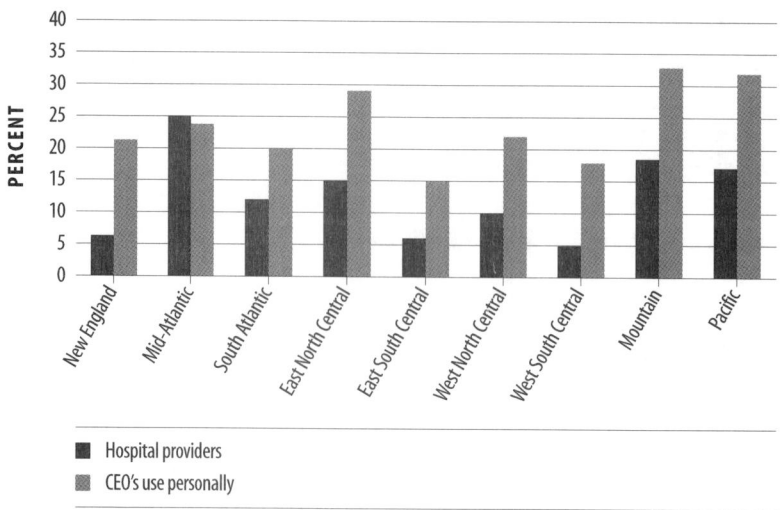

■ Hospital providers
■ CEO's use personally

reimbursement, scope of practice and access to CAM providers. For example, Washington state law now mandates coverage for CAM.

Most hospitals still do not grant privileges to alternative medicine providers, although the percentage varies greatly with size and location of the facility. According to a survey by the American Hospital Association, 10.2 percent of the 552 hospitals surveyed in 1999 are offering some form of complementary medicine, up from 7.7 percent in 1998 (Modern Healthcare, December 4, 2000, p. 8). Ironically, somewhere between 15 to 35 percent of hospital chief executive officers surveyed by Deloitte & Touche do use some form of complementary medicine (U.S. Hospitals and the Future of Health Care, 2000) (See Figure 8). Still, the infrastructure for learning about and providing complementary care is limited, while the acceptance of complementary care among healthcare providers, and even some consumers, varies greatly by age, region, and other demographic and socioeconomic characteristics.

Strategic Implications for Healthcare Organizations
1. If present trends continue, an increasing number of hospitals and healthcare providers will begin to offer CAM techniques. In the long run, to be sustainable, these services must either positively contribute to bottom line or demonstrably enhance the organization's value proposition to the marketplace.

2. Studies on CAM will continue to verify its effectiveness. As scientific evidence mounts to support the efficacy of select modalities of complementary care, such modalities will be gradually accepted by "allopathic" medicine.

3. Healthcare organizations that make no effort to accommodate or integrate alternative medicine techniques run the risk of not only missing a market opportunity, but also alienating an expanding segment of the population.

Strategic Implications for Health Information Technology Organizations
As CAM is adopted by more healthcare providers, HIT systems will ultimately need to ensure that systems can accommodate these new modalities of care. This will include the requirement that the systems possess the requisite lexicon unique to CAM.

Barriers
1. Though as many as 60 percent of all Western, therapeutic interventions cannot be explained using a scientific model, the prevailing allopathic paradigm is so strong and pervasive as to form a potent barrier for the integration of complementary modalities.
2. The lack of reimbursement by most insurance plans will continue to hinder the integration of many complementary services into many care processes.

Section 2.0 – Technology/E-Strategy

2.1 Electronic Medical Records/Clinical Information Systems

Background

Despite the immense promise of advanced information technologies (IT) generally and the electronic medical record (EMR) in particular, integrated IT systems have been slow to take root in the healthcare market. Few dispute the contention that patient-centric information systems can transform healthcare by creating a more efficient, paperless environment, which, among other things, would allow for true portability of health information. However, evidence suggests that adopters are still few and far between. According to the 2001 HIMSS Leadership Survey, only 13 percent of senior executives and managers of healthcare organizations report that they have a "fully operational" EMR in place. More than 25 percent have not even begun to plan for implementing such a system. And just 3 percent of the 550,000 doctors in private practice in the United States use EMRs, according to Cary, North Carolina-based A4 Health Systems, while only one-tenth of one percent of physicians have gone fully paperless (See Figure 9).

The reasons for dismal EMR adoption rates include technological or operational shortcomings with the systems themselves, severe and ongoing financial constraints among providers, as well as an aversion to change on the part of users.

On the technology front, many products are designed to focus on only one piece of the delivery model, whether it is the administrative or clinical side, while some systems concentrate on just one component of administration or clinical care, such as lab, pharmacy or billing. The failure to provide a user-friendly interface through which data can be accessed, the lack of integration with legacy information systems, limited

Figure 9. Computer-based Patient Record System Usage
Source: 11th Annual HIMSS Leadership Survey, 2000.

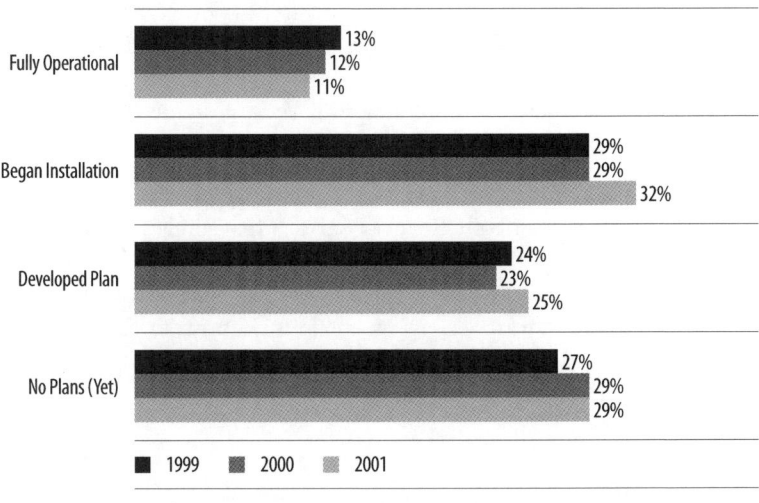

Figure 10. Top Concerns for Security of Computer-based Medical Information
Source: 11th Annual HIMSS Leadership Survey, 2000.

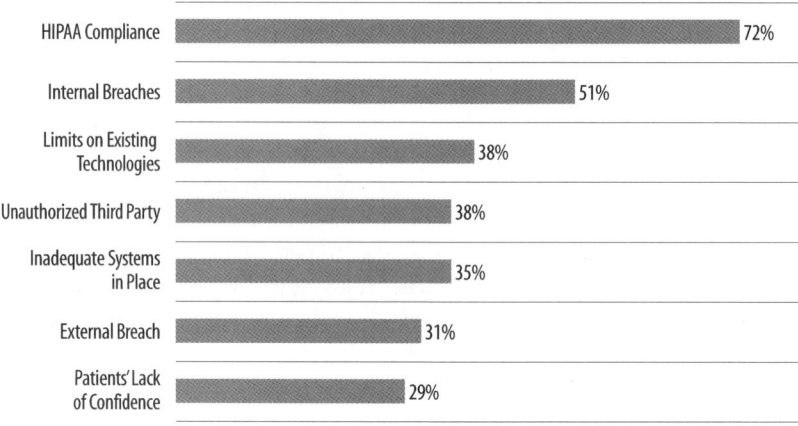

off-site access, sporadic or non-existent after-acquisition training and support, and organizations' needs for real-time data likewise have contributed to the disappointing adoption rate.

Separately, the issues of HIPAA compliance, internal security and unauthorized use of electronic information as they relate to the EMR are major concerns for health executives (HIMSS Leadership Survey, 2000) (See Figure 10).

Many health information technology companies are beginning to break down some barriers by providing more fully integrated solutions, as well as portable or flexible interfaces that include voice recognition software, handheld wireless devices and web-based applications that use Internet protocols to enable information to be more easily exchanged.

Efforts are also underway to create standards for defining the interface requirements of systems throughout the healthcare system, although a single, preferred architecture for the EMR has yet to emerge. Regardless of the architecture eventually settled upon, it must be able to receive data feeds from all points of care for the EMR to be of optimal value. Such points of care range from physicians' offices to ambulatory diagnostic facilities to inpatient settings. Accomplishing this level of connectivity between disparate settings will be challenging.

That said, addressing the technological impediments to widespread EMR deployment may prove easier than reducing the financial barriers that hinder greater implementation. At present, most healthcare organizations continue to feel the sting of major Medicare reimbursement reductions triggered by the Balanced Budget Act of 1996. In addition, uncompensated care levels in many regions continue to rise, as do the costs of labor, medication and other clinical inputs. Many long-time players consider the current financial environment among the most challenging ever in the history of the modern healthcare industry.

Allocating capital for costly IT systems consequently is a low priority for many institutions, particularly those struggling to survive. Moreover, proving the return on investment (ROI) of EMR implementation is not a straightforward process, primarily because of the large variation in core processes across providers. As such, attempts by technology companies to support ROI assertions with data have, at best, only limited applicability and relevance to many healthcare organizations.

The emergence of Internet-based application service providers (ASPs) does offer the promise of less-costly IT solutions, particularly for smaller, rural facilities. By outsourcing their IT requirements through a remotely located vendor and accessing the system via the Internet, hospitals can reduce capital and maintenance expense while still enjoying the benefits of a robust EMR. However, hospitals effectively relinquish control of their network with the ASP model and are therefore critically dependent on the vendor for system reliability, maintenance and security.

In spite of the obstacles, adopting advanced information technologies does produce a wide range of benefits that can dramatically improve quality of care as well as internal operational systems and processes. Just a few of these benefits include:
- Improved clinical documentation
- Improved customer service
- More efficient clinical workflow
- Improved medication management
- Decreased chart pulls
- Fewer lost charts
- Better communication between providers
- Reduced transcription costs
- Reduced labor costs

One of the most promising trends in healthcare information technology has been the development of next-generation EMRs that incorporate decision-support capabilities into the systems. This type of functionality allows providers and other organizations to practice evidence-based medicine by delivering knowledge at the point of care and monitoring results in real-time.

Decision support and expert systems ultimately will help providers constantly refine their definitions of what constitute "best practices" by analyzing treatment patterns and outcomes over a large patient population. In addition, as consumers, employers and payers begin to demand validation of the quality and value of providers' healthcare services, organizations will have a compelling need for the outcomes information generated by the EMR.

One major healthcare IT issue that remains unsettled is who should own and have access to the information contained within the EMR. The Health Insurance Portability and Accountability Act (HIPAA) was written to address some of these concerns; however, the ultimate ownership issue has not been resolved. Many believe that consumers are the only ones who have a truly vested interest in effectively managing their own healthcare information. Certainly, empowering consumers with their own health information would, for better or worse, accelerate the trend toward self-guided care.

Skeptics, however, maintain that patients are not qualified to oversee their own care and consequently should not be provided with the tools to do it. At the same time, providers maintain that allowing patients to control their health information would be cumbersome and could thwart the timely delivery of care.

Other countries are facing this issue and developing unique responses to the question of medical information ownership. In France, consumers are being issued healthcare smartcards, which are essentially credit cards containing microprocessors that store and process portions of an individual's health record. The United States, however, is far from even contemplating such a model.

Strategic Implications for Healthcare Organizations
1. Despite what is arguably the most difficult financial environment ever in healthcare, providers must find ways to generate and allocate capital for investment in the deployment of electronic medical records and other advanced healthcare information technologies.

2. Providers must not lose sight of the fact that the EMR and attendant information connectivity across all points of care provide real solutions to many of the systemic problems that plague healthcare today, including operational inefficiencies, wide variances in care and the prevalence of medical errors.

3. Healthcare providers will need to overcome the inertia that often thwarts innovation in the delivery of care to embrace a cultural transformation that places a major emphasis on improved customer service, improved operational efficiency and a reduction in both medical error and care variation.

4. Health systems that deploy EMRs and other advanced information technology must make the protection of patient information a top priority and must work diligently to implement mandates of HIPAA, however vague, lest consumers and government leaders lose faith in healthcare's ability to prevent the abuse of electronic medical information.

Strategic Implications for Health Information Technology Organizations
1. Healthcare IT organizations must generate cost-benefit studies that clearly and unequivocally demonstrate the return on investment that EMR systems provide.

2. Healthcare IT organizations need to work closely with providers to develop incentivized payment schemes that take into account both the current economic challenges facing providers as well as the historic skepticism that many providers hold toward lavish IT benefit claims. Furthermore, HIT organizations must lobby alongside healthcare organizations for increased reimbursements for the use of technology.

3. New applications must be capable of interfacing with legacy information systems to preserve the significant investment many organizations have already made in older IT technology. Furthermore, IT systems must be developed which support the seamless integration of patient information across the entire continuum of care and across disparate IT products.

4. Training and ongoing application supports need to be primary components in IT hardware-software proposals to ensure the system is optimally used and delivers on cost-benefit promises.

5. Developers of ASP-model EMRs must be particularly attentive to the need for in-depth, redundant system safeguards that eliminate the possibility of even partial system failure. They also must stress unmatched client service and support in their product offerings. This approach will help reduce the reluctance many health organizations have to entrusting mission-critical information systems to remote, external providers.

6. While many HIPAA security standards can be met through existing EMR systems, HIT organizations must continue to design products with HIPAA compliance in mind.

2.2 Changing Role of the Chief Information Officer

Background

Just as information technology has been elevated to the mainstream in healthcare, so too has the profile of the chief information officer (CIO) within the healthcare organization. Increasingly the CIO is moving away from an operations-based role associated with IT systems infrastructure, support and acquisition, and evolving into a legitimate executive role as strategist and facilitator of organizational success. At the same time, the traditional executive team comprising the chief executive officer (CEO), chief operating officer (COO) and chief financial officer (CFO) is becoming savvier of the role IT systems play in achieving organizational success. In fact, as a leadership survey conducted by the Healthcare Information and Management Systems Society (HIMSS) demonstrates, members of the executive team constitute more than 75 percent of primary non-IT sponsors for IT projects (See Figure 11).

In light of the executive team's heightened awareness that IT is a key enabler of strategic objectives, as well as the magnitude of new IT investments, the CIO can expect a shift away from his traditional role of systems and hardware acquisition. The CIO will no longer need to be the sole organizational flag bearer of IT, encouraging its use and broad integration into daily operations. Rather, his role will lie with making the busi-

Figure 11. Who Is The Primary Non-IT Sponsor For IT Projects In Your Organization?
Source: 11th Annual HIMSS Leadership Survey, 2000 — provider responses.

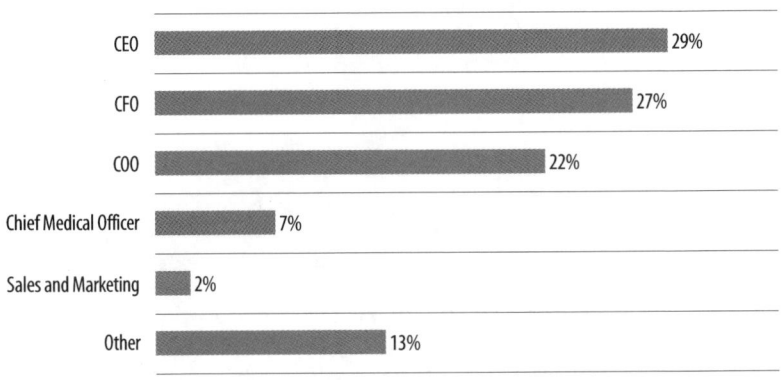

Figure 12. Percent of IT Spending Controlled Outside IT Department (n=486)
Source: 12th Annual HIMSS Leadership Survey, 2001 – provider responses.

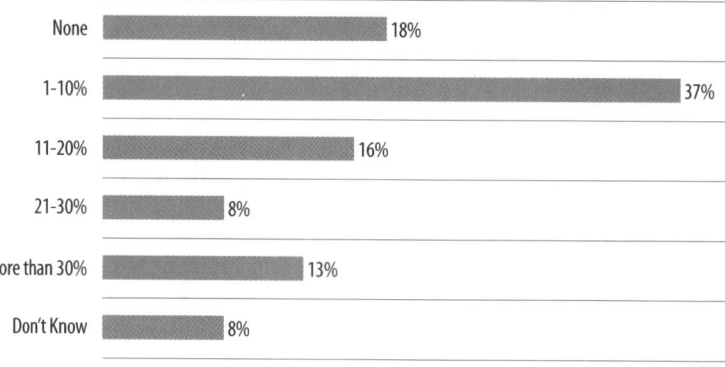

ness case for targeted IT initiatives, so as to empower the entire executive team to make purchasing decisions consistent with organizational strategy. A prime example is in the area of enterprise resource management solutions, technology designed to achieve the maximum return from the supply chain and other operational areas – clearly a function falling within the purview of the CFO. While it will remain imperative that the CIO have input into such acquisition decisions, his role will for the most part lie with making the business case for targeted IT initiatives, specifically as it relates to ROI and competitive differentiation. As such, the CIO will continue to play a key role in IT acquisition decisions, yet can expect to see a greater percentage of IT spending being controlled outside of the IT department, primarily by the executive team (See Figure 12).

Strategic Implications for Healthcare Organizations
1. The role of the CIO in healthcare organizations will continue to move away from that of IT support and operations and into the domain of strategic leadership. As such, the CIO must be fully recognized as a legitimate member of the senior executive team.
2. Within the context of organizational strategy, the CIO must develop the business skills necessary to communicate IT imperatives to the executive team, including:
   - Return on investment from efficiencies realized and the ability to "do more with less"; and
   - Competitive differentiation through improved quality, patient safety and staff satisfaction.

Strategic Implications for Health Information Technology Organizations
1. Technology vendors that are able to provide a business case for their products, supported by ROI information validated through primary research, will significantly differentiate themselves from competitors.
2. Technology vendors must broaden their marketing efforts to include a target audience composed of the entire executive team, including the CEO, COO, CFO and CIO.

2.3 E-business Capabilities

Background

IT not only contributes to the actual delivery of care, but it also supports finance and administrative processes as well. While the EMR is arguably the foundation of a comprehensive IT strategy, various healthcare entities including hospitals, health plans and vendors are increasingly shifting process-management systems to Internet platforms. In fact, according to a survey by *Computer Economics,* spending on e-commerce software by hospitals increased more than 47 percent during the first half of 2000.

In the earliest days of the Internet revolution, much of the activity was centered on the development of passive content, or so-called "brochure-ware." Hospitals were quick to create Web sites that advertised their services, although most were unable to leverage these sites to improve revenues. Third-party content providers such as drkoop.com also emerged, targeting consumers seeking healthcare information. While consumers may have profited from these initial endeavors (see section 1.2 on the rise of consumerism), organizations did not. In fact, last year drkoop.com laid off 55 percent of its staff and its long-term sustainability remains questionable. Other early entrants into the content arena, such as WebMD, increasingly have identified non-content revenue streams to drive profitability.

Most recently, much of the focus in healthcare e-commerce has been on business-to-business transactions designed to automate and streamline the healthcare supply chain. Either through traditional group purchasing organizations or new purchasing portals, hospitals are now ordering a small but growing volume of materials through the Internet.

According to Millennium Research Group, online purchases of medical supplies increased steadily through the second half of 2000 to 3.5 percent of total volume by October, up from 2.6 percent of total volume in June 2000. The overall market for hospital medical materials is estimated at about $100 billion. Observers believe that $11 billion of that expense could be eliminated through Internet-driven improvements in supply chain purchasing and inventory management. Most observers anticipate that Internet procurement in healthcare will grow rapidly over the next two years, reaching 47 percent of all medical equipment and supply purchases by 2003.

Leading e-procurement providers like medibuy and Neoforma.com have thus far weathered the Internet shakeout and continue to add customer volume through acquisitions or alliances. At the same time, 2000 saw the formation of the Global Healthcare Exchange, a consortium of five of the world's leading medical products manufacturers. This initiative, which added four more medical suppliers in late 2000 and whose members collectively sell to 90 percent of the hospitals worldwide through traditional means, promises to be a force in the e-healthcare supply chain industry going forward.

Beyond the high level of activity in the supply chain arena, other sectors of healthcare e-business remain in their infancy. As a result of the large number of disparate parties involved in the financing and delivery of healthcare, the Internet does offer enormous potential for transaction support and connectivity. The technology that will contribute to a connected marketplace includes the Internet, intranets, extranets, application service providers and legacy systems. In some areas, health plans already are using the Internet to automate business processes that involve providers and consumers, including referrals, authorizations, claims, eligibility and reporting.

In Florida, for example, Blue Cross and Blue Shield of Florida and Humana have joined forces to create an Internet portal that physicians can use to automate routine administrative functions, such as checking referrals or submitting claims.

Connectivity between and among providers also holds considerable promise. Hospitals and providers are benefiting from increasing communication with colleagues, largely by transmitting lab results and other patient information. Approximately 55 percent of physicians use e-mail to communicate with other professionals, although only 14 percent currently interact with patients via e-mail. According to a survey by the Health Technology Center, diagnostic reporting topped the list of applications that physicians believe the Web can be most effective in delivering, followed by claims processing and pharmaceutical information. Emerging capabilities that demand multi-player connectivity include the scheduling of appointments, the transmission of test results to patients and the renewal of prescriptions online.

In Atlanta, Children's Healthcare recently debuted a Web portal that allows doctors to access clinical and demographic information via a secure Internet connection tied to the hospital's intranet. Using the system, physicians can access patient histories and physicals, X-ray reports, pending orders, lab results, discharge summaries and consults.

Because most healthcare organizations do not have the capital to implement numerous e-business capabilities, the strategies to be adopted next and those that are maintained will be the ones that create efficiencies, enhance revenues or reduce costs. E-business has the potential to increase the levels of customization and customer loyalty, as well as the speed with which information is shared. Knowing this, healthcare organizations will continue to try to find ways to leverage technology to gain a competitive advantage.

Strategic Implications for Healthcare Organizations

1. Providers should determine which of their processes could most effectively be automated with the greatest return on investment and then begin the process of migrating those services to a Web platform. The range of possibilities includes eligibility, claims, referrals and authorizations, as well as systems for peer-to-peer communication.

2. Because supply chain automation offers real cost benefits, providers should likewise shift all or some of their purchasing to one of the many e-procurement organizations. Since most of the traditional group purchasing organizations have developed some form of Internet procurement capability, shifting to the Web does not necessarily mean severing long-standing ties with existing organizations.

3. Capital must be identified and planning must begin for the development of the infrastructure necessary to provide ubiquitous Internet connectivity across healthcare organizations. Whether PC or wireless, or a combination of both, this infras-

tructure will be necessary to accommodate the surge of Web-based healthcare applications looming just over the horizon.

4. Healthcare organizations may want to consider partnering with competitors or other organizations to develop truly community-wide Internet healthcare connectivity. While this approach would necessarily be complex, the "first-mover" benefits that would accrue in the marketplace would likely make the effort worthwhile.

5. Healthcare providers must adopt business-to-business (B2B) and business-to-consumer (B2C) interoperability standards to facilitate a wide range of information transactions made possible by the proliferation of the Internet. Interoperability standards adoption will serve to virtually integrate once disparate stakeholders, including consumers, providers, health plans and payers and healthcare product vendors. Such integration will facilitate improved access, efficiency and reliability throughout the health system.

Strategic Implications for Health Information Technology Organizations

1. A survey of physicians conducted by the Health Technology Center found that 93 percent considered "the lack of system compatibility across healthcare organizations" to be a critical barrier to realization of the full potential of Internet-enabled systems in medicine. It is therefore incumbent upon the industry to work toward interoperability standards that promote communication across the entire care spectrum.

2. Internet applications or services that produce a demonstrable and immediate return on investment, either through revenue enhancement or cost reduction, offer the greatest likelihood of success for vendors, given the economic realities in healthcare today.

3. Partnerships or alliances that combine domain knowledge and expertise from a variety of areas have proven effective for many Internet companies in more quickly achieving critical mass in a highly competitive marketplace.

2.4 Telemedicine/Telehealth

Background

Telemedicine, or telehealth, relies on video and telecommunications technology – sometimes coupled with robotics – to transmit diagnostic images, conduct interactive videoconferences, provide health assessments and garner second opinions. Telemedicine also provides a unique platform for interactive distance learning opportunities for both patients and clinicians. Since emerging in the 1970s, telemedicine's most common uses have been in the educational area, as well as in the enhancement of healthcare services in rural areas. Applications are becoming more ubiquitous, however, and increasingly are being deployed in urban settings. The University of Maryland Medical Center in Baltimore, for instance, now uses ambulance-based video and computer technology to assess the condition of stroke victims as they are being transported to the hospital.

Widespread adoption of telemedicine historically has been limited by a range of factors, including high costs, bandwidth concerns, government regulation, lack of government and private payer reimbursement, unclear return on investment, lack of image transmission standards and providers' cultural resistance to change. Yet some of these barriers are beginning to fall, and most experts anticipate that advances in information technology will contribute to substantial growth in the demand for telemedicine products and services in the years just ahead (See Figure 13). Currently, approximately 85 percent of healthcare organizations in 32 states are using one or more telehealth applications. (Health Care 2000, p. 151) (See Figure 14).

Figure 13. U.S. Market for Telematics
Source: Telemedicine Opportunities for Medical and Electronics Providers. Business Communications Company, 1998.

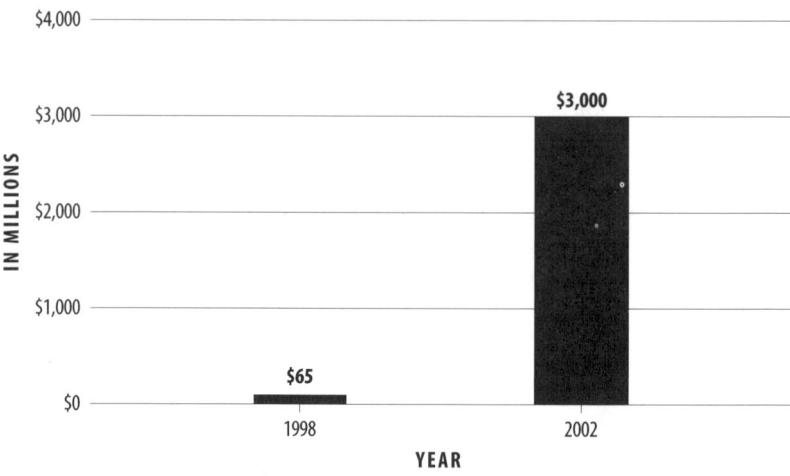

Figure 14. Telehealth Applications in Use by Healthcare Organizations
Source: 10th Annual HIMSS Leadership Survey, 1999.

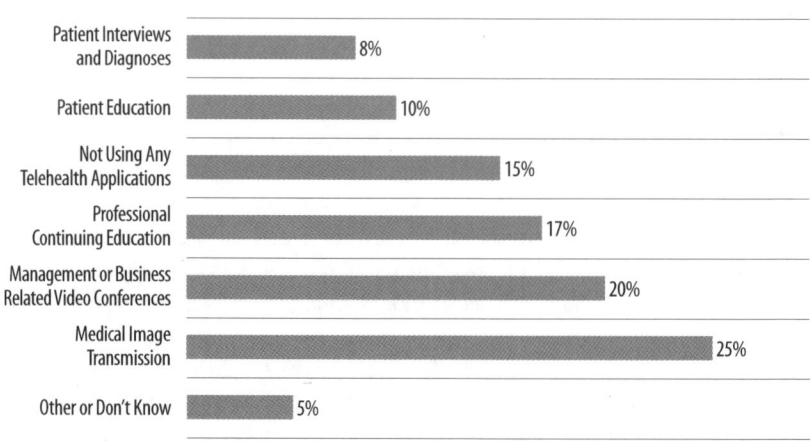

The growth of telemedicine will be fueled to a great extent by the unprecedented functionality and connectivity offered by the Internet, which will significantly reduce the cost of services. At the same time, the expanding presence of broadband connectivity, including fiber optics, DSL and cable, is allowing for far faster and larger text, voice, image and video media transmissions across the Web.

Telemedicine is also benefiting from decisions by the primary government payers – Medicare and Medicaid – to reimburse certain telemedicine services for beneficiaries in medically underserved areas. Some of these reimbursed services include radiology, some prisoner healthcare, psychiatry and home healthcare.

At the same time, the complex patchwork of differing state laws that govern the delivery of care across state boundaries is slowly being updated to accommodate a digital world. At present, three states have passed reciprocal licensure laws, which provide a simplified application process and lower licensure fees for telemedicine practitioners. Organizations like the Federation of State Medical Boards of the United States and the American Medical Association have drafted comprehensive model regulations and are working to have them adopted.

One of the most promising areas of telemedicine involves the interpretation, storage and retrieval of digital images, including x-rays, MRI images and CT scans. Dramatic increases in the volume of clinical imaging – now growing at about 13 percent per year in the United States – combined with a growing shortage of radiologists, is forcing an increasing number of providers to rely on outsourced, remote radiology services accessed through the Internet. This trend is expected to accelerate rapidly in 2002 as a result of a decision five years ago that effectively increased the residency requirements for radiologists-in-training from four years to five. As a result, virtually no new radiologists will enter the job market next year and the shortage of practicing radiologists will become acute.

On a separate front, the ability to aggregate a wide range of digital images via telemedicine holds significant promise in the area of diagnosis improvement. For example, an Atlanta-based firm, Medizeus Inc., has developed software aimed at improving the accuracy of mammogram screening from approximately 85 percent today to the low 90s. The software, which measures a patient mammogram against a library of digitized images showing confirmed malignancies, becomes more "intelligent" by incorporating each new image into its memory and is therefore capable of generating more effective and accurate comparisons with each use.

Providing consultative services in rural areas underserved by conventional healthcare resources is, and will likely remain, perhaps the most attractive applications of telemedicine. The benefits included quicker consultations, greater access to a wider range of expertise and reductions in travel expense and risk for patients, particularly elderly individuals compelled to travel great distances in adverse winter conditions.

In South Dakota, Avera St. Luke's Hospital in Aberdeen provides a range of telemedicine services for 15 rural hospitals and clinics that are representative of the kinds of programs presently being implemented in rural areas. These services include wellness programs, such as dietary consulting, smoking secession and diabetic support for patients, as well as continuing medical education for rural healthcare staff in a variety of disciplines.

Telemedicine also holds promise in the urban setting. Charles R. Drew University in Los Angeles last year opened its third urban telemedicine site in an effort to improve access to healthcare for inner-city residents. The facilities currently provide pediatric care and ophthalmology services to several thousand patients.

Going forward, telemedicine promises to provide the ability to remotely and continually monitor patients with chronic illnesses, as well as opportunities afforded for remote testing and treatments using robotics. Ultimately, the increasing use of telemedicine will result in patients requiring fewer face-to-face encounters with their physicians. In addition, telemedicine has the ability to increase access and encourage more widespread prevention and screening practices.

Impediments remain, however, not the least of which are the mixed results of cost-benefit analyses regarding telemedicine. The number of studies that have fully investigated the financial benefits of telemedicine at present is too small to be able to generalize about their conclusions, although some studies have suggested that certain types of telemedicine programs may be quite cost-effective, especially those that avert transportation costs or create out-of-area referrals.

In rural areas, the relative scarcity of broadband connections continues to hamper more widespread use of telemedicine. At the same time, the lack of a simple, universally deployable electronic medical record has impeded the adoption of telemedicine. Documentation of telemedicine consultations will be cumbersome and complicated if a paper-based record remains the dominant mode of recording and storing medical information. With electronic records, health information and relevant images from telemedicine consultants can easily be aggregated into a dispersible, multimedia patient record.

Strategic Implications for Healthcare Organizations
1. Healthcare organizations should identify operational areas or programs that could be well served via telemedicine and work to inform payers about the economic benefits these programs could provide.

2. Providers likewise should align with national and state advocacy groups to hasten the adoption of uniform state licensure laws that will allow for greater flexibility in the practice of telemedicine.

3. Telecommunications upgrades, whether to accommodate telemedicine or an expanding Internet presence, are critically important for providers that seek to remain competitive over the next five to ten years.

Strategic Implications for Health Information Technology Organizations
1. Technology should readily support remote communications requirements, be they videoconferencing or consults, remote radiology readings or distance learning.

2. Technology vendors should create a range of demonstration sites highlighting the capabilities of telemedicine and showing that it can be just as effective – and considerably cheaper – than the face-to-face delivery of care.

Section 3.0 – Scientific/Clinical Trends

3.1 Advances in Genomics and Biotechnology

Background

Biotechnology is a discipline that combines molecular biology, recombinant chemistry, genomics, proteomics, drug development, and information technology to create new approaches in the detection and treatment of diseases. Of all the environmental factors identified heretofore, advances in biotechnology promise to have the most profound long-term impact on the provision of healthcare in America.

Much of that change will be driven by genomics, or the study of genes and how they function. In 2000, scientists associated with the Human Genome Project and with Celera Genomics, a private corporation, independently completed a "working draft" of the human genome sequence. This goal was achieved years ahead of schedule as a result of advances in technology. The identification of the more than 30,000 genes in human DNA creates a wealth of possibilities for the future of medicine that promise to transform many aspects of healthcare. Among the genomics-based therapies now emerging:

- **Gene testing** allows clinicians to test individuals for the presence of genetic material that may predispose that individual to a particular disease state. So far, genetic tests have been developed for a range of conditions, including cystic fibrosis, glaucoma, colon cancer and inherited kidney diseases. In addition, prenatal gene testing also is available for Down's syndrome and certain birth defects.
- **Gene therapy** involves the introduction of new DNA into a patient to repair or replace a defective gene. Currently, more than half of the early clinical trials in this area target some form of cancer.
- **Synthetic proteins** are being developed to augment or replace proteins created by malfunctioning genetic material. Synthetic or recombinant proteins currently are available to treat a number of disease states, including hemophilia, prostate cancer, myocardial infarction, chronic anemia, multiple sclerosis, rheumatoid arthritis and hepatitis C.
- **Individualized drugs** customized to match the genetic predisposition of the patient hold the promise of both improving efficacy through more refined dosage levels and reducing the risk of adverse drug events through the identification of previously hidden genetic defects or anomalies.

Proteomics, which focuses on the role of proteins and their interactions within the body, is another arena of rising importance. Proteins are manufactured by genes to execute the specific instructions of the genes within the body. Hence, they are major players in the development of disease and ultimately may provide even more detailed clues to the manifestation of disease than genes. Celera is just one of several companies conducting studies in the field of proteomics and has raised more than $983 million in capital to continue research in this area. It is probable that more companies and resources will be dedicated to proteomic research and development in years ahead.

The implications of the genomics and proteomics revolutions are profound, if not yet crystal clear. Genomics may well trigger a fundamental shift in healthcare from its current focus on treating disease to preventing it. Most experts believe that for many disease states, genomics will result in earlier diagnosis, as well as faster, cheaper and more effective treatments. At the same time, the emphasis on prevention and early detection will alter healthcare's current focus on intervention from middle age or old age toward the prenatal period or childhood. This will include a growing reliance on screening would-be parents for genetic deficiencies or vulnerabilities. Care increasingly will transpire in outpatient settings through non-invasive therapies. Genomics also will likely lead to more standardized, evidence-based medicine grounded in rigorous scientific research.

Most healthcare executives believe that genomics – particularly genetic mapping, or the development of detailed genetic databases on individuals, a prerequisite for genomic therapy – will increase the costs of care (See Figure 15). However, it is not at all clear to what extent payers will be willing to absorb these costs, since insurance companies historically have been less inclined to pay for preventive care than for after-the-fact procedures and treatments.

Although considerable enthusiasm has been generated in the equity markets about the prospects of pharmcogenomics, or the development of new medications designed to take advantage of genomic advances, the costs of developing these drugs will likely be significant in the near-term. A study by Lehman Brothers and McKinsey & Co. concluded that the average research and development costs of bringing a new chemical entity (NCE) to market will increase from about $800 million today to between $1.3 billion and $1.6 billion by 2005. The increase is attributed to the wider range of possible target compounds presented in the genomics environment, along with the initial absence of empirical information about pharmacogenomic processes with respect to a specific compound.

Figure 15. Percentage of Respondents Who Agreed Strongly That Genetic Mapping Would Result in These Outcomes
Source: HealthCast 2020, PricewaterhouseCoopers.

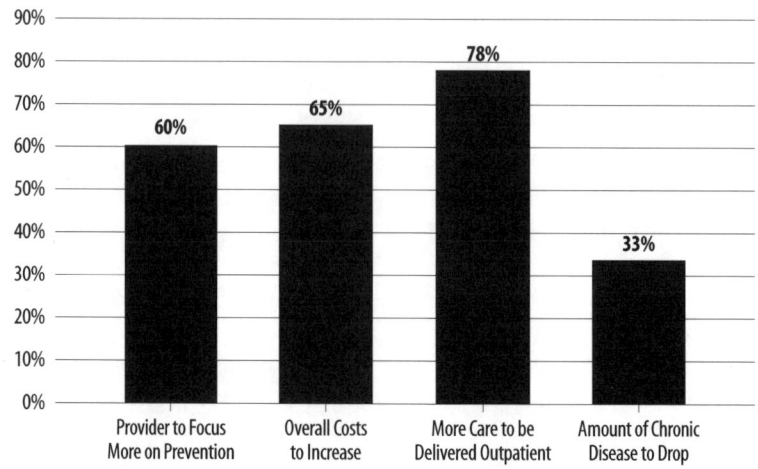

Nonetheless, pharmacogenomics unquestionably will produce an enormous number of new, highly effective drugs. These will include so-called "designer drugs" formulated to minimize adverse reactions while working with a person's genetic make-up or with other drugs that an individual may be taking. Screening methods could also be tailored to individuals and diseases. Pharmaceutical firms are partnering with biotechnology companies to advance these areas of research.

On a separate front, the curriculums of medical schools will necessarily be required to incorporate a growing thread of genomics across all disciplines, and clinical genetic specialists will emerge, particularly in the area of pediatrics, since many tests will begin in childhood. As genomic therapies become more commonplace and their benefits more widely publicized, competition among providers will likely become intense. Those healthcare organizations that make early efforts to develop genomic capabilities likely will be rewarded; those that delay could pay a significant price in the marketplace. Already, a Genomics Task Force created by the Mayo Clinic has recommended an investment of between $50 million and $100 million in resources to help the organization capture an early leadership position in the arena of genomics-based medicine.

The clinical and delivery implications of genomics, while immense, are at least equaled by the legal and ethical issues that have emerged with the discipline. For example, the prospect that genomics will help increase the average lifespan to 95 over the next 50 years raises difficult questions about the wisdom of extending life for individuals whose conditions would otherwise cause them to die sooner. Chief among these concerns is the possibility that these individuals would reproduce and, in so doing, perpetuate a genetic flaw or anomaly to the next generation. In general, providers must be prepared to address the profound ethical impact genomics will have on reproductive decision-making and rights.

At the same time, creating genetic profiles on individuals increases the possibility that employers or insurance companies would use the information to deny employment or coverage for individuals whose make-up showed a predisposition to a disease that was particularly expensive to treat. Separately, the ability to identify a genetic predisposition to a disease for which there is no cure begs questions about the psychological impact this information could have on the individual.

Another potential problem is the likelihood that many genomic therapies may be available only to those with the most generous health plans, or those willing to pay for the therapies out-of-pocket. This possibility raises the prospect of an emerging "genetic underclass" as described by Myers, et al., for whom the genomics revolution will remain out of reach.

In addition, serious issues of liability surround genomics. One key question involves the obligation of physicians to perform genetic testing, or genotyping, on an individual once such testing becomes widespread. Theoretically, the physician could be liable if genetic testing would have revealed a specific condition or pre-condition, or if it would have precluded or prevented a complication, particularly as it related to prescription of medications by the attending doctor. Other areas of potential liability include privacy issues surrounding access to genetic information, as well as safety issues associated with the development of novel drugs or treatments.

Some of these issues were brought into focus in 1999, when a patient at the University of Pennsylvania Health System died after being treated with an experimental genomic therapy designed to address a mild form of liver disease. A lawsuit filed by the 18-year-old's parents alleged that the patient was not a proper study subject because of abnormal test results, and that he had not been properly informed about the risks associated with the experimental treatment. As a result of the tragedy, the University of Pennsylvania closed its gene therapy program.

Information technology will play an important role in the further advancement of biotechnology. Bioinformatics is the use of computers and information technology to acquire, store and analyze biological data, which is often in the form of large, complex information data sets.

Bioinformatics is an area of "sophisticated analytical tools, number-crunching computers, whole laboratories on wet chips, DNA chips, combinatorial chemistry chips and a host of sci-fi technology that are automating research tasks" (Healthcare Informatics, January 1999). Bioinformatics relies not only on software advancements but also improvements in hardware, such as advanced chip technology. Additionally, computer simulations, data mining and high through-put screening capabilities will be used to assist in the development of new medical technologies, with the result likely to be reductions in research and development costs.

Major computer companies, such as IBM and Compaq, are entering the bioinformatics market and creating hardware and software programs to help analyze the complex information being generated by biotech research. IBM is building super computers and in December 2000 sold the world's largest commercial computer to a genomic research firm.

Continued development in the areas of genomics and biotechnology will depend on increased funding for research and development. The cost and time required to develop and bring a technology or genomic application to market is great, and support in the past has primarily come from the government or Wall Street. By June 2000, the market capitalization of the biotech industry had increased 156 percent from the previous year. Additionally, initial public offerings for biotech companies have been averaging about $100 million per offering, which is significantly higher than in past years. The total investment in biotechnology in the form of initial public offerings, venture capital and financing rounds was approximately $35 billion in 2000. However, only a small percentage of biotechnology companies achieve profitability. A primary revenue source for biotechs is selling information from their genome databases or gene chips. The strong stock performance of these firms also reflects the possibilities of being acquired by large pharmaceutical corporations.

Consumers have welcomed the application of medical technologies and genomics to disease prevention and treatment, despite their hesitance to embrace other applications such as cloning and genetically engineered foods. When new gene testing and other therapies do become widely available, it is assumed that consumers will want access to them immediately and will expect their health insurance to pay for them. Unfortunately, it is likely that such applications will be expensive. Consequently, the stage will be set for exacerbated conflict between consumers and healthcare payers.

Consumers will also demand that the result of any genetic testing be protected and not used for discrimination purposes. While HIPAA will address the privacy and security of personalized medical information, specific provisions will need to be written to address the sanctity of genetic information. As a result, encryption technology and authentication software could become increasingly important.

Strategic Implications for Healthcare Organizations
1. Providers need to closely monitor clinical developments in genomics and begin assessing the potential cost-benefit-demand picture for services that are likely to emerge or gather momentum in the next several years. Adding genomic therapies to service offerings will require that providers strike a balance between the premature pursuit of unproven treatments and tardy or grudging acceptance of demonstrably beneficial therapies. Those organizations that choose to ignore the clinical and operational implications of genomics will do so at their peril.

2. Providers must work with trade organizations and other advocacy groups to begin developing ethical and legal guidelines for genomic therapies. Chief among these considerations will be privacy considerations surrounding a patient's genetic profile.

3. Similarly, providers need to explore the global cost-benefit implications of genomics, perhaps through joint analysis with payers, to help foster a reimbursement environment that takes into account the potentially enormous savings that effective preventive medicine could generate.

Strategic Implications for Health Information Technology Organizations
1. The explosion of genomic research is creating demand for bioinformatics-oriented hardware and software (Healthcare Informatics, Body Language, 1999). Those companies able to leverage existing competencies in this area stand to benefit significantly.

2. Developers of clinical information technologies for provider organizations must begin assessing the growing role genomics will play in medicine. Likely requirements that a genomic-centric delivery system will require include the collection, storage, transfer, security and access of individual genetic records.

3.2 Improving Quality of Care and Patient Safety

Background

Although quality is important in any industry, in healthcare it can make the difference between life and death. The prestigious Institute of Medicine has released two reports specifically addressing the issues of medical error and healthcare quality. The first report, released in 1999 and entitled *To Err is Human: Building a Safer Health System*, suggested that as many as 98,000 deaths occur each year related to medical errors – primarily because of poorly designed systems of care (See Figures 16 & 17). The second report, released in 2001 and entitled *Crossing the Quality Chasm: A New Health System for the 21st Century*, lays the conceptual framework for the fundamental

Figure 16. Most Commonly Reported Types of Medical Errors
Source: Leape L, et al. "The Nature of Adverse Events in Hospitalized Patients."
New England Journal of Medicine, 324 (6), 1991.

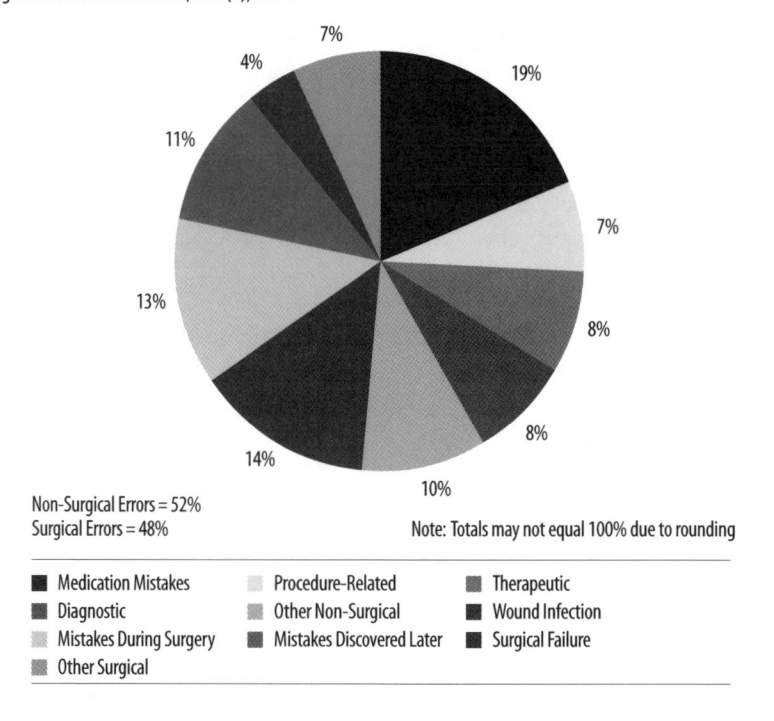

Non-Surgical Errors = 52%
Surgical Errors = 48%

Note: Totals may not equal 100% due to rounding

- Medication Mistakes
- Diagnostic
- Mistakes During Surgery
- Other Surgical
- Procedure-Related
- Other Non-Surgical
- Mistakes Discovered Later
- Therapeutic
- Wound Infection
- Surgical Failure

Figure 17. Preventable Medical Errors
Source: Leape L, et al. "Preventing Medical Injury." Quality Review Bulletin, 19 (5), 1999.

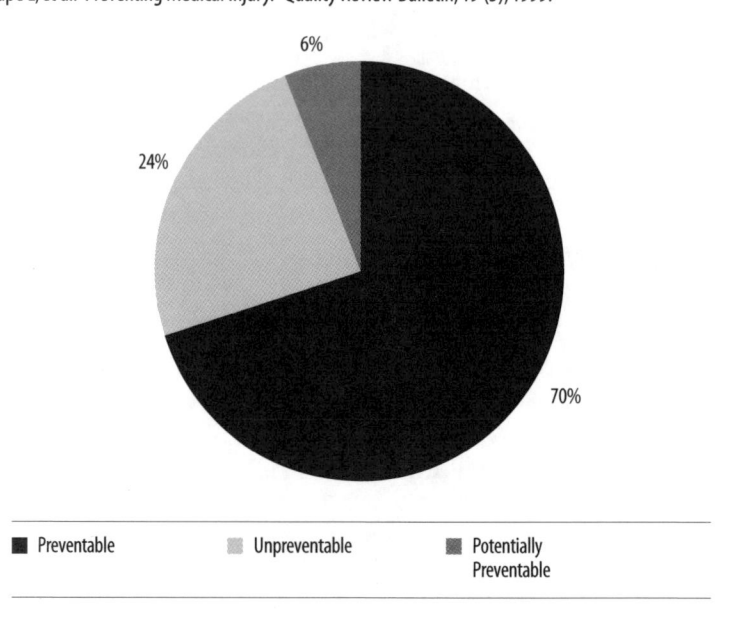

- Preventable
- Unpreventable
- Potentially Preventable

redesign of the U.S. healthcare system, at the heart of which lies strong recommendations for the proliferation of evidence-based medicine and the use of clinical information systems.

The government, along with individual organizations, has begun to devote substantial resources to studying the problems of medical errors and healthcare quality. Additionally, the business community, through organizations like the Leapfrog Group, has tried to use the IOM Reports as catalysts for improving the quality, safety and value of care provided for its employee benefit dollars. The Leapfrog Group is attempting to use the combined purchasing power of its members to mandate the adoption of clear standards of quality as a prerequisite for payer contracting.

The reasons to devote resources to reducing medical error are numerous, with the most important being to save lives. In addition, although the number of studies is small, quantitative evidence does exist to support the assertion that reducing medical errors will result in cost savings for provider organizations. For example, errors associated with medications represent the largest classification of medical errors. The estimated cost of a medication error is $2,500 to $3,500 per bed per year. In a 300-bed hospital, eliminating medication errors could translate into more than $1 million savings in just one year. An even larger potential for savings exists if errors are reduced in the ambulatory settings (Futurescan 2001). The IOM report *To Err is Human* estimated that medical errors could cost the U.S. healthcare system between $17 billion and $29 billion each year.

The healthcare system does have some mechanisms already in place to promote the delivery of quality healthcare. Healthcare providers have long been subject to regulations and accreditation requirements aimed at this objective. The Joint Commission on the Accreditation of Healthcare Organizations has as its mission to "continuously improve the safety and quality of care to the public." The National Committee for Quality Assurance aims to "evaluate and report on the quality of the nation's managed care organizations." Other important organizations, such as the Health Care Financing Administration, state agencies and a host of other entities, place healthcare organizations under continuous scrutiny. Unfortunately, it could be argued that these organizations have not been effective at improving the quality of healthcare. Numerous research studies spanning a period of two decades have clearly documented the prevalence and magnitude of quality concerns, and specifically medical errors. Yet, in many cases, the provider community has not aggressively acted on the results of these studies and has in some cases even adopted the perspective that quality problems do not exist at their facilities.

Currently very little information is available to the public about healthcare quality. "Report cards" or quality rankings are beginning to be published specifically for consumers, and they already serve as popular information sources for those who are looking for the best provider or facility to treat a specific condition. Although most consumers are not able to dissect the methodology behind these ratings, they do value the information. But how often and to what extent the information affects choices and

Figure 18. Proportion Who Have Seen Any Information Comparing the Quality of Health Care Plans, Doctors, or Hospitals Within the Last Year
Source: Kaiser Family Foundation/Agency for Health Care Policy and Research/Princeton Survey Research Associates, Americans as Health Care Consumers: The Role of Quality Information, October, 1996.

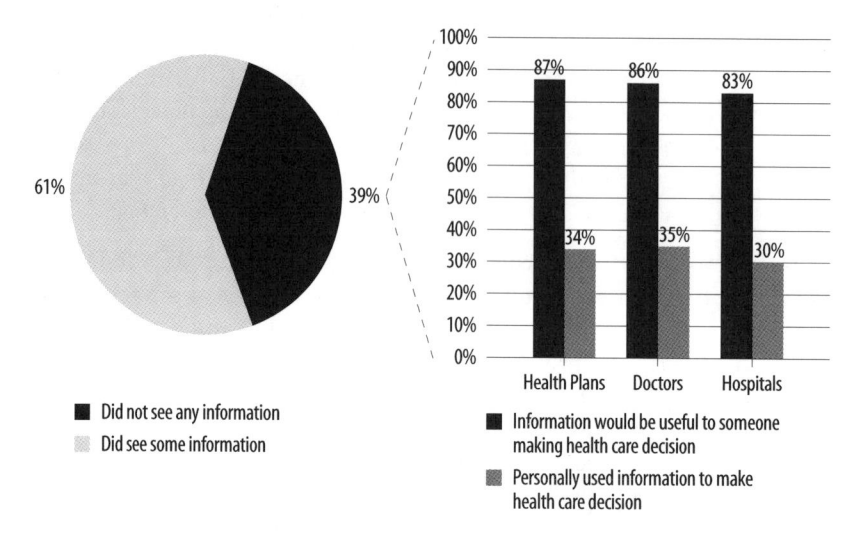

- Did not see any information
- Did see some information
- Information would be useful to someone making health care decision
- Personally used information to make health care decision

decision-making is not well known. The Kaiser Family Foundation investigated the role of quality information and found that some consumers are actually using information in decision-making but many are not (See Figure 18).

For example, the Health Plan Employer Data and Information Set (HEDIS) measures – used to rate the quality and performance of health maintenance organizations – have not been as widely utilized by employers or consumers as was initially predicted. In 1997, only 24 percent of employers indicated that HEDIS data played a role in their health plan decision-making process (Center for Studying Health System Change, 1998, p. 79).

Providers often are skeptical of how healthcare rankings are determined and question their validity. The information sources used to create these rankings vary from survey to survey and few actually compare provider performance against generally accepted clinical benchmarks. Yet providers do not readily dismiss these systems, primarily because consumers find these rating systems useful. In fact, providers who are recognized in reputable rankings often leverage that exposure as a marketing opportunity.

Currently, a private sector-based group, the Washington, D.C.-based National Quality Forum, is working to develop standardized metrics that will accommodate valid quality comparisons across all healthcare organizations. The forum includes representatives of government and business, as well as provider and consumer groups, and is targeting summer of 2001 for the completion of a preliminary strategy for national quality benchmarks.

The greatest potential for improving the quality of healthcare, especially with regard to the reduction of medical error, may surround advances in information technology. Applications such as computer alert systems, computerized physician order entry and decision-support systems promise to enhance the provision of care. For example, a computer alert system implemented at Banner Health in Phoenix, Ariz., identified opportunities to reduce adverse drug events at a rate of 64 per 1,000 admissions (JAMA 1998: Vol. 280, 1317-1320). At Brigham and Women's Hospital in Boston, a computerized physician order entry system reduced medical errors by 55 percent. Unfortunately, despite the promise of technology in reducing medical error, providers have not embraced these solutions. Some of the greatest barriers appear to be lack of capital, competing priorities and the inability of new systems to interface with existing systems (See section 2.1 on computerized medical record). Overcoming these barriers will be difficult but necessary for the potential benefits of technology to be realized.

Whether or not the momentum associated with the current focus on healthcare quality can be sustained remains to be seen. Although the fragmentation of the current healthcare delivery model complicates the provision of consistent, high-quality care, opportunities for improvement clearly exist. However, it is likely that it will take continued and increased pressure from consumers, employers, the government and other advocacy groups to truly impact the quality of care.

Strategic Implications for Healthcare Organizations

1. The complacency that has marked many providers' reaction to the publicity surrounding medical error must be replaced with an aggressive and sustained commitment to improving the quality of care. Failure to do so could result in a significant diminution in the trust and goodwill the U.S. health system has accumulated over decades, not to mention expansive liability.

2. Reducing variations in care through standardization – either evidence-based medicine or strict treatment protocols – are options that can have an immediate and meaningful impact on medical error. Physician reluctance to follow treatment protocols should not be a roadblock to implementation of such programs and procedures.

3. Information technology holds enormous promise for reducing medical error. Whether used to provide easier access to accurate medical records, for decision support or to track and measure outcomes, HIT provides effective solutions for mitigating error and improving quality. Healthcare organizations must embrace the technological advances that other industries have used for years to improve efficiency and quality.

4. Providers should seek opportunities to participate in reputable rankings and help consumers understand what those rankings mean. Even though the criteria for determining performance may differ from one ranking to the next, healthcare providers and organizations should identify ranking institutions and seek to achieve exceptional performance based on the existing criteria. They should also support the adoption of national benchmarks through which performance can be measured.

Strategic Implications for Health Information Technology Organizations

1. HIT vendors should stress the impact that existing information systems can have on medical error, while continuing to refine the development of applications that assist in the reporting and prevention of medical errors.

2. Information technology companies should develop rigorous cost-benefit case studies that demonstrate the financial benefits that can result from the reduction of medical error through IT solutions.

3. Vendors should partner with provider organizations to lobby for increased reimbursement and/or the development of financial incentives for reducing medical error. Under the current payment scheme, providers have little direct incentive for reducing error, although the indirect financial benefits can be significant.

4. Perhaps collectively through trade organizations, vendors should sponsor rankings, awards or other mechanisms for recognizing healthcare organizations that have effectively implemented information technology.

5. HIT organizations should support standards initiatives that promote the cost-effective integration of new and legacy information systems.

Section 4.0 – Government/Regulation

4.1 HIPAA/Privacy/Security Regulations

Background

In the mid-1990s, much attention was given to a piece of legislation informally referred to as the Kennedy Kassebaum bill. At that time, the focus of the bill was on guaranteeing continuous insurance coverage to individuals (regardless of preexisting conditions) who may be compelled to switch insurance carriers as a result of changing jobs. The bill was passed in August 1996 and was named the Health Insurance Portability and Accountability Act (HIPAA).

One section of the act initially received minimal attention but is now creating significant anxiety for healthcare administrators and providers. The section, entitled Administrative Simplification, established guidelines to "reduce the costs and administrative burdens of healthcare by making possible the standardized, electronic transmission of many administrative and financial transactions that are currently carried out manually on paper" (HCFA, 1997). The specific components of this section of the law include standards for:

- The privacy of electronic health information
- The security of that information
- Electronic data interchange (EDI) transactions
- The use of unique health identifiers for each individual, employer, health plan, and provider.

Of all the proposed standards, it is the privacy regulations that have generated the most attention and emerged as an area of significant concern for both consumers and healthcare organizations. Consumers advocate that the most stringent measures should be taken to protect their medical information from unauthorized use. On the other hand, healthcare providers are worried about their ability to guarantee such levels of privacy.

Now that the final privacy standards have been released, healthcare organizations, clearinghouses, providers and plans have two years to implement them. Doing so will have a significant impact on these organizations. Some of the greatest concerns are related to the extensive requirements for compliance, the cost associated with implementation and timeframes for implementation. The Department of Health and Human Services estimates total implementation costs to be $3.2 billion for the first year and almost $18 billion over the next ten years. However, other estimates project up to $43 billion over five years (Healthcare Business, March 2001). Information technology executives find it hard to predict what the actual costs will be (See Figure 19).

HIPAA compliance will require organization-wide effort, as well as cultural and behavioral changes within healthcare organizations. Despite its far-reaching impact, only 29 percent of senior hospital managers consider themselves to be very knowledgeable about the regulations. Almost 80 percent said it is a top business issue in the next two years, but 23 percent have not yet begun to plan for it (12th Annual HIMSS

Figure 19. Percent of CIOs Who Believe That HIPAA Expenses Will Be:
Source: Healthcare 2000, page 134.

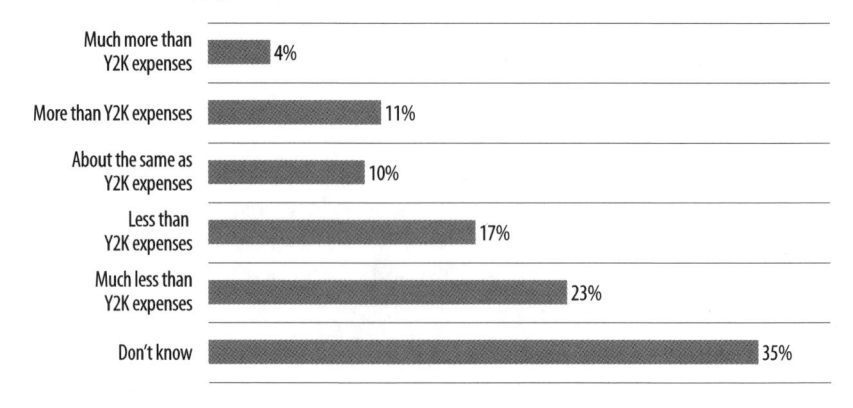

Much more than Y2K expenses	4%
More than Y2K expenses	11%
About the same as Y2K expenses	10%
Less than Y2K expenses	17%
Much less than Y2K expenses	23%
Don't know	35%

Figure 20. Actions Taken to Achieve HIPAA Compliance
Source: 12th Annual HIMSS Leadership Survey, 2001

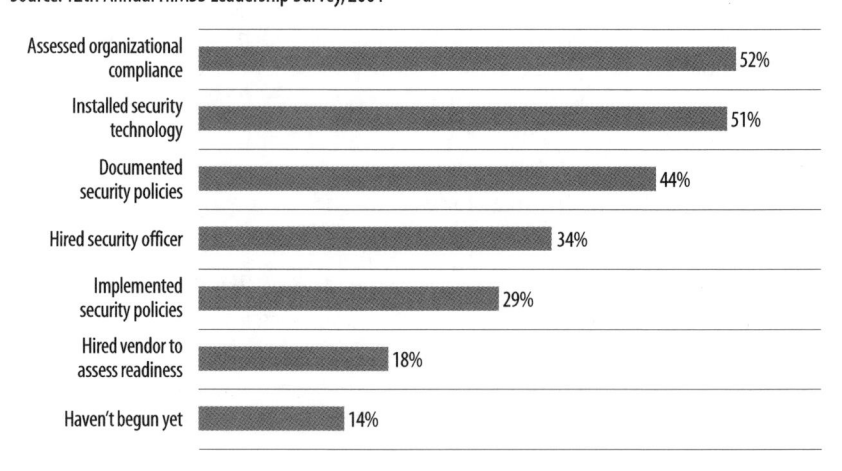

Assessed organizational compliance	52%
Installed security technology	51%
Documented security policies	44%
Hired security officer	34%
Implemented security policies	29%
Hired vendor to assess readiness	18%
Haven't begun yet	14%

Leadership Survey, 2001). The steps that most organizations have been taking to prepare for HIPAA are outlined in Figure 20.

Of the few organizations that are well on the road to compliance, many report that conducting a comprehensive assessment of the organization and educating employees contribute most to the successful implementation of compliance strategies (Hospitals and Health Networks, February 2001, p. 39). Additionally, ensuring the support of senior management and business partners also is important. Although the short-term costs and time requirements for HIPAA compliance will be great, the savings that could be achieved as a result of improved efficiency in the electronic transfer of information and business practices could be worth billions of dollars in the long run.

Strategic Implications for Healthcare Organizations

1. However onerous the task may appear in light of the associated costs, healthcare organizations should develop comprehensive strategies for achieving compliance that incorporate all aspects of the organization. Furthermore, healthcare organizations must create systems for appropriate process redesign, staff training, and ongoing monitoring and compliance.

2. This will require particularly rigorous training and education for compliance staff to ensure that the organization remains abreast of the latest changes or modifications in the statutes.

3. Organizations should view HIPAA not as a threat, but as an opportunity to modernize information systems and move toward full automation of many back-office functions that traditionally have been labor-intensive, error-prone and inefficient. Those organizations able to quickly capitalize on the greater provider-payer-patient connectivity that HIPAA will allow should reap significant benefits, both in reduced costs and improved customer service.

Strategic Implications for Health Information Technology Organizations

1. Helping provider organizations become HIPAA-compliant represents a sizable consultative market opportunity. Components of a typical compliance strategy will include assessment of current systems and level of compliance, remediation of areas not in compliance, and implementation of new systems and processes. As such, HIPAA compliance efforts may create a synergistic opportunity for consultants and HIT vendors to partner in helping healthcare organizations become compliant.

2. The next several years will present opportunities not only to market HIPAA-specific applications, but also to effectively demonstrate to providers the need for significantly upgraded IT capabilities.

3. Improving the functionality of technical compliance solutions, including data encryption devices, biometrics and the like, will give vendors an opportunity to differentiate themselves in a crowded IT marketplace.

4.2 Regulation of Drug Costs

Background

In 1998, the annual prescription drug expenditures in the United States were $93.4 billion and accounted for almost 10 percent of the total U.S. healthcare spending. For health plans, drug costs account for 12 to 15 percent of their overall costs and could increase to 20 percent in the next few years (Center for Studying Health System Change, 1999). Both the average cost per prescription and drug utilization have been increasing (See Figure 21). In fact, pharmaceutical costs rose 16.9 percent in 1999 and 17.4 percent in 2000 (Modern Healthcare, March 12, 2001, p. 15). These growth rates far exceed the increases seen in other areas of healthcare spending. In 1999, the average cost of a prescription drug was $71.49, more than twice the average cost of $30.47 for drugs introduced before 1992, according a study produced by the National Institute of Health Care Management.

Figure 21. Growth in Prescription Drug Expenditures
Source: Factors Affecting the Growth of Prescription Drug Expenditures. Prepared by Barents Group, LLC, for the National Institute for Health Care Management Foundation, July 1999.

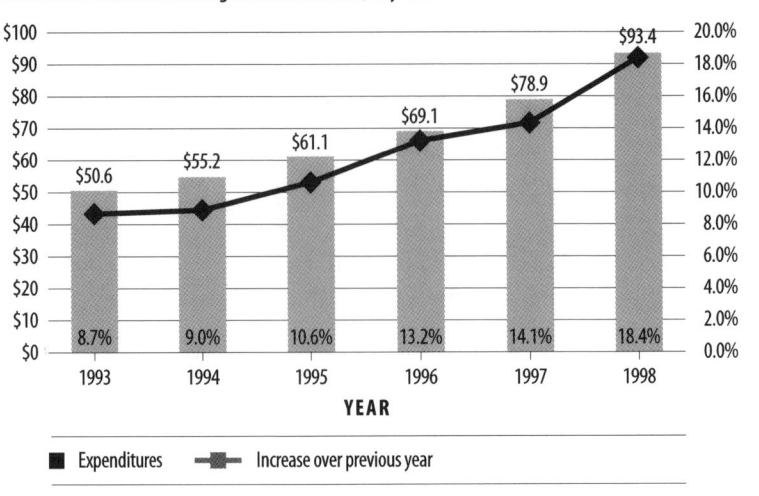

Year	Expenditures	Increase over previous year
1993	$50.6	8.7%
1994	$55.2	9.0%
1995	$61.1	10.6%
1996	$69.1	13.2%
1997	$78.9	14.1%
1998	$93.4	18.4%

Pharmaceutical companies maintain that high costs for drugs are the result of the significant investments that must be made in research and development. In 1999, pharmaceutical companies spent about $24 billion on new drug development and improving current products. Moreover, as drug companies point out, only a small fraction of drugs developed and tested actually make it to market. According to the Pharmaceutical Research and Manufacturers of America, it takes 12 to 15 years and approximately $500 million to discover and develop a new drug. Furthermore, only one in 5,000 to 10,000 compounds screened eventually becomes an approved drug (Pharmaceutical Research and Manufacturers of America, *The Value of Pharmaceuticals*).

Supporters of price regulation acknowledge that while these facts are accurate, pharmaceutical companies also spend large sums (more than $2 billion in 2000) for marketing directly to consumers and physicians and deliver healthy dividends to shareholders. The ten most-advertised medications accounted for approximately 22 percent of the total increase in prescription drug costs between 1993 and 1998 (Health Care, 2000, p. 31). Given the controversy surrounding increasing drug prices, pharmaceutical companies and their practices will continue to receive close scrutiny.

According to a survey by Harris Interactive, public satisfaction with the pharmaceutical industry has dropped 13 percent in the last year (Petersen, 2000). Most consumers now have to pay more out of their personal income for medications, as Medicare and health maintenance organizations decrease drug benefits, and commercial insurers introduce three-tier co-payments. Consumers want the newest, most effective and often most expensive drugs available and are unwilling to go without their medication unless they have no other choice. Unfortunately, many seniors do not have the financial resources to pay for their medications themselves and consequently must do without.

Consumer groups and the federal and state governments are beginning to take action aimed at reducing drug costs. Some states have already begun to regulate drug prices and the federal government is investigating price controls in relation to Medicare reform (see Section 6.1). The likelihood of success for these efforts is difficult to forecast, although it is clear that pharmaceutical companies will aggressively fight restrictive regulations.

For pharmaceutical companies to effectively thwart price controls, they must be able to demonstrate, in financial terms, the value that pharmaceuticals generate in terms of improved outcomes, illness prevention and the elimination or reduction of cost-intensive clinical treatments. Although these benefits are extremely significant, many observers believe the industry has failed to effectively illuminate or quantify the gains in dollar terms. Consequently, it is important that pharmaceuticals gain access to data that would allow them to clearly demonstrate the relative cost-effectiveness of medications versus clinical alternatives. Doing so would help drug companies price products more effectively and possibly reduce the clamor for price controls.

Going forward, pharmacogenomics, or the development of drugs that act on advances in genetics, promises to create an enormous range of new benefits for patients, although medications will likely be costly in the near-term (See Section 3.1). At the same time, the prospect of more than $30 billion worth of brand-name drugs coming off patent by 2005 will create significant opportunities for generic drug manufacturers and should contribute to reduced costs for some of the nation's most popular and effective drugs.

Strategic Implications for Healthcare Organizations
1. Because pharmaceutical companies will aggressively resist any benefit mandates that do not fully compensate the drug producers, healthcare providers likely will remain caught between rising drug prices and patients clamoring for the latest and best medications.

2. Three-tier health plan formularies that require enrollees to pay more out-of-pocket expense if they choose a branded drug over an equivalent generic continue to evolve as a means of controlling medication costs. Essentially, formularies shift the burden of cost-benefit decisions from the health plan to the patient.

3. A greater awareness of generic drugs by providers – particularly physicians – could help arrest soaring medication costs. The prospect of a dramatic increase in the number of available generics should boost usage over the next decade.

Strategic Implications for Health Information Technology Organizations
HIT organizations can expect an increasing market for IT products that enable remote study monitoring, provide for rapid data analysis, and otherwise reduce pharmaceutical research and development costs and time to market. While it may be naïve to assume that pharmaceutical companies will pass these savings on to consumers, HIT organizations nevertheless stand to profit significantly from such applications.

Section 5.0 – Economic/Reimbursement Trends

5.1 Healthcare Costs Increase

Background

More than $1 trillion is spent on healthcare in the United States each year. Approximately 60 percent of this amount is consumed by hospital care, physician services, pharmaceuticals and other medical non-durables. Over the past decade, total healthcare costs have accounted for 13 to 14 percent of the gross domestic product. However, it is likely that this figure will rise to 16 to 17 percent in the next few years. The Health Care Financing Administration reported that healthcare spending grew 8.3 percent in 2000, and they project increases of 7.1 percent in 2001 and 9.9 percent in 2002 (Modern Healthcare, March 12, 2001, p. 5) (See Figures 22, 23, & 24).

A period of relative cost stabilization in healthcare between the late 1980s and the late 1990s was largely attributable to the growth of managed care and government regulation (for example, the Balanced Budget Act of 1997). The introduction of utilization management, different payment methodologies and reduced payment rates to providers all played significant roles in keeping costs down. However, healthcare provider and consumer backlash has more recently exposed the limits of government and managed care firms' ability to contain medical costs. Many managed care companies have posted unprofitable quarters or years of late and, as a result, are seeking to increase premiums while developing less controversial methods of managing their members' medical care.

Whether or not the economy continues to prosper will be an important factor in healthcare spending. Expenditures for healthcare tend to increase at a higher rate than

Figure 22. National Healthcare Expenditures
Source: Health Care Financing Administration, Office of the Actuary, Division of National Health Statistics, 7500 Security Blvd., Baltimore, MD 21244, www.hcfa.gov

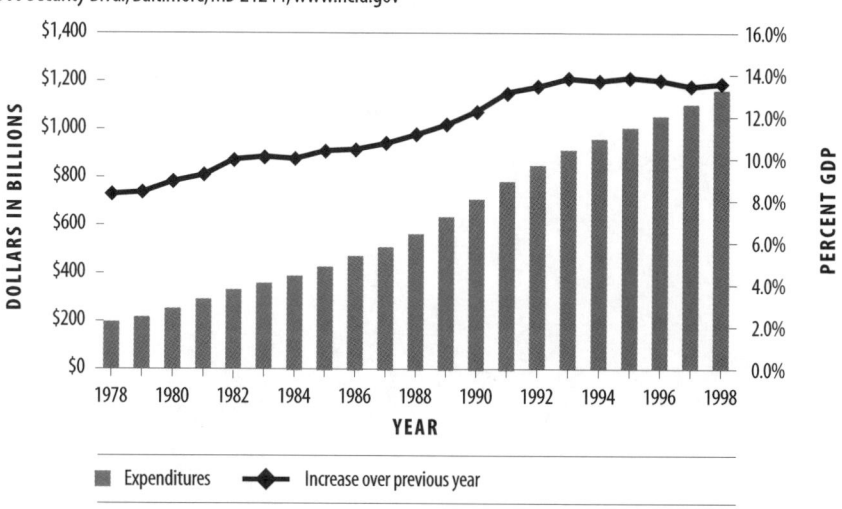

Figure 23. National Health Expenditures "Services and Supplies" 1998–2000
Source: "Health Affairs" March/April 2001

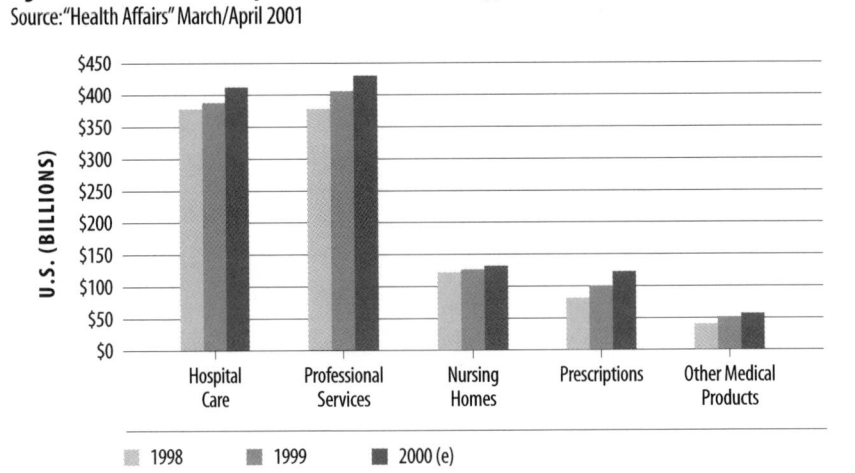

Figure 24. Medical Inflation
Source: US Labor Dept., Bureau of Labor & Statistics, Economic Analysis & Information, 230 S. Dearborn Parkway, 9th Floor, Chicago, IL 60604.

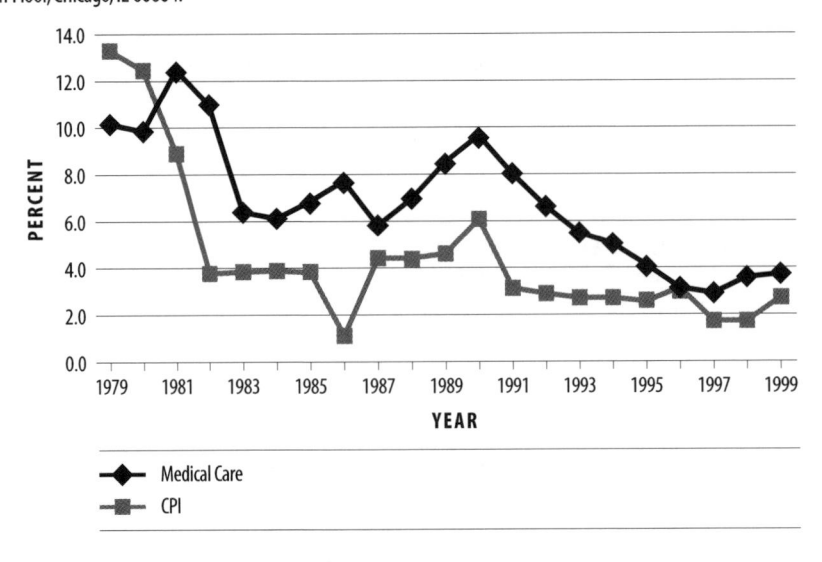

other types of spending during a recession. Uncertainty about job stability and future insurance availability drives up utilization and cost (PricewaterhouseCoopers, Healthcast 2010, 1999, p. 26). Consequently, further economic downturn will push spending to higher rates. At the same time, the aging population, as a result of their increasing demands for health services, also will drive spending up.

Strategic Implications for Healthcare Organizations

1. In light of pressure from the government and third-party payers to reduce costs, healthcare organizations must seek to eliminate current inefficiencies in the delivery of care through systems redesign.

2. Real-time performance information in such critical areas as utilization management, clinical outcomes and supply chain management will be a key enabler of cost-reduction strategies as providers mobilize to meet the challenges of external cost-containment pressures.

3. As consumers become less insulated from the cost of healthcare through increased premiums and out-of-pocket expenses, they will increasingly seek the highest value for their healthcare dollar. As such, providers that are able and choose to proactively provide consumers with data relative to quality and cost along clearly defined value metrics stand to significantly differentiate themselves from competitors.

4. HIT will be a fundamental enabler of healthcare cost reduction strategies in the long run, despite the initial and significant up-front investment organizations will be required to make.

Strategic Implications for Health Information Technology Organizations

1. Cost-containment strategies aimed at healthcare organizations will ultimately result in diminished capital reserves for major expenditures. With that in mind, HIT vendors will be challenged to develop creative purchasing arrangements to accommodate the limited capital funds of the majority of healthcare providers.

2. HIT organizations must tailor implementations to be quick and cost-effective so healthcare organizations can almost immediately begin to realize a return on investment.

3. Information systems must be designed to support the instantaneous transfer of clinical information from multiple feeds into a comprehensive operations picture of an organization.

5.2 Financial Instability of Healthcare Organizations

Background

Healthcare organizations are pressured to deliver high-quality care at a low cost. Meeting this mandate has become increasingly difficult. Examples of organizations that encountered serious financial problems – such as Allegheny Health System and Harvard Pilgrim Healthcare – are increasingly prevalent. The American Hospital Association reported that almost half of U.S. hospitals produced a profit margin below 3 percent in 1999, which is even below the rate of medical inflation (Modern Healthcare, December 2, 2000). More than 50 percent of HMOs reported losses in 1997 and 1998 (Health Care, 2000, p. 85). By 2002, it is possible that profit margins of hospitals could fall as low as 0.041 percent (Ernst & Young/HCIA). Although some relief was delivered to providers and health plans by the Balanced Budget Refinement Act (BBRA) and the Benefits Improvement and Protection Act of 2000 (BIPA), the majority of healthcare organizations continue to struggle financially. If profit margins are not improved, more bankruptcies of healthcare organizations could occur.

Escalating cost structures, increased competition and inefficient systems, processes and management, as well as anemic reimbursements from both public and private payers are contributing to diminished profitability for healthcare organizations. Organizations are responding by implementing financial improvement initiatives, which include analyzing the services they deliver and selecting only those that are the most profitable to market and expand (See Figure 25). Some organizations have even

Figure 25. Services with the Greatest Increase and Decrease in Investment by Percentage
Source: American Hospital Association's Health Forum, 1999.

Services with the Greatest Increase in Investment by Percentage	
Trauma	18.6%
Case Management	13.6%
Urgent Care	9.7%
Positron Emission Tomography	9.4%
Magnetic Resonance Imaging	9.1%
Cardiac Cath Lab	8.7%
Crisis Prevention	8.1%
Occupational Health Services	7.4%
Women's Health Services	7.3%
Angioplasty	7.1%

Services with the Greatest Decrease in Investment by Percentage	
Transplant Services	-40.5%
Other Long-Term Care	-37.4%
Other Care	-22.0%
Other Special Care	-18.0%
Retirement Housing	-17.6%
Other Intensive Care	-12.3%
Assisted Living	-11.0%
Adult Day Care Program	-10.4%
Reproductive Health Services	-9.8%
Home Health Services	-6.9%

adopted niche strategies. Not surprisingly, these specialty organizations are considered a threat to many full-service providers because their success is predicated upon their ability to provide services that do not require the full and expensive infrastructure of a tertiary inpatient setting. Typically, these organizations build their own consumer-friendly, ambulatory care settings and deliver care at these facilities. The theory of the niche providers is similar to that proposed by Regina Herzlinger in her book *Market-Driven Healthcare*. Herzlinger argues that organizations should focus on a set of core competencies and deliver them to a narrowly defined customer segment. Examples of niche players include HealthSouth, MedCath and US Oncology. These for-profit organizations typically seek to deliver select services that offer favorable reimbursement.

A common strategy that healthcare organizations are adopting to improve financial performance is the pursuit of market share gain. Hospitals and systems are attempting to compensate for lower reimbursement by increasing volumes. These efforts have been supported by increases in both inpatient and outpatient admissions. In 1999, inpatient cases rose by 1.7 percent, while the number of outpatient visits increased 4.4 percent.

Improving profit margins will continue to be an area of critical importance for the majority of healthcare organizations. Those that are not able to generate moderate margins will be unable to attract investors or capital to maintain their infrastructure. Small hospitals, particularly in rural areas, will be most impacted by the recent trends of rising costs and declining reimbursement. Unfortunately, no evidence exists that this trend will turn around anytime soon. In 1999, the average adjusted cost of an inpatient admission increased 2 percent to $6,512, but revenue per adjusted admission rose only 0.7 percent (Modern Healthcare, December 4, 2000 p. 2).

One of the reasons profit margins of many healthcare organizations have stayed positive, despite numerous pressures, has been the contribution of investment income (See Figure 26).

Figure 26. Hospitals Post Another Profitable Year
Source: Hospital Statistics, American Hospital Association, One North Franklin Street, Chicago, IL 60606

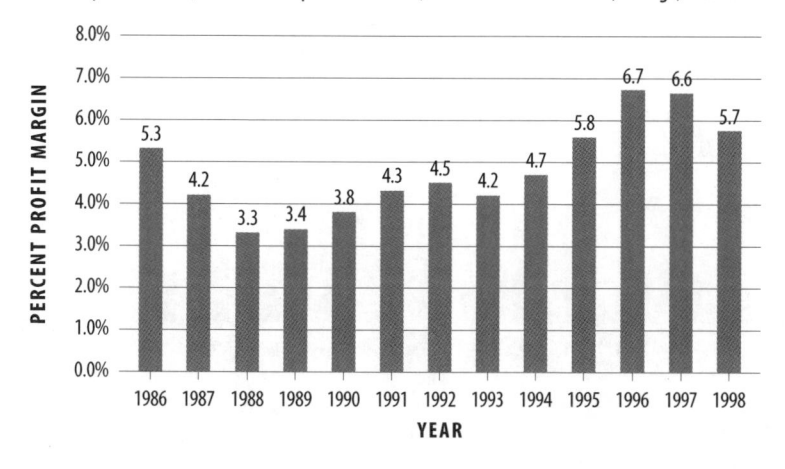

In 1998, a survey of hospitals who received an "A" rating from Standard & Poors indicated that 60 percent of these hospitals' total margin was derived from investment income (Modern Healthcare, December, 2000). Unfortunately, the recent volatility of the equity and bond markets suggests that future investment income may be lower than in previous years and, as a result, profits may fall. In addition, many not-for-profit hospitals have experienced bond-rating downgrades (See Figure 27). Both Moody's Investor Services and Standard & Poors, however, in early 2001 forecasted more stable bond ratings by the end of the year, even though the number of downgrades will continue to outpace the number of upgrades. Moody's also changed its rating of the for-profit hospital industry sector from negative to stable as a result of a less volatile Medicare market, increased admissions and improved reimbursement from managed care companies.

Strategic Implications for Healthcare Organizations

1. Providers must focus on expanding operations or services that are profitable and reducing or eliminating those that are not. While this approach admittedly runs counter to traditional concepts of comprehensive, mission-driven healthcare, today's economic realities no longer afford providers the luxury of attempting to be all things to all people.

2. Proactive cost management is necessary to effectively operate in the current environment. Process reengineering, benchmarking and the adoption of best practices are vital for economic survival in the long run.

3. Any plan to significantly enhance the performance and efficiency of a healthcare organization arguably must begin with an information infrastructure capable of automating many processes now done manually. Assessing internal IT needs and examining vendor capabilities is a starting point for organizations committed to long-term improvements.

Figure 27. BBA Leads to Bond-Rating Downgrades for Not-for-Profit Hospitals
Source: Moody's Investors Service, 2000.

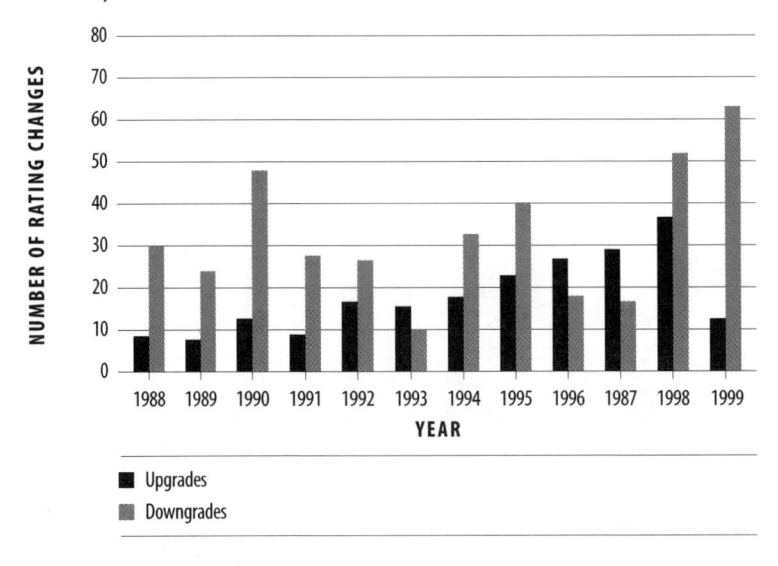

Strategic Implications for Health Information Technology Organizations
1. Capital available to invest in new technology will be limited. Consequently, if healthcare providers are to adopt technology, they will do so only if it provides a compelling and demonstrable return on investment.
2. Vendors need to find new ways to reduce financial barriers that limit the adoption of information technology.

5.3 Emergence of New Financing Models

Background
The structure of the financing and delivery model for healthcare in the United States creates conflict between the various participants, as well as inefficiency and ineffectiveness. Though the United States spends more dollars per capita on healthcare than any other nation in the world, it consistently ranks far below virtually all other developed nations in terms of the care delivered to its populace. In fact, in a study by the World Health Organization published in June 2000, the effectiveness of the U.S. healthcare system ranked 37th in the world.

The misaligned priorities of physicians, hospitals, payers, employers and consumers contribute to the system's ineffectiveness. Employees are seeking coverage for the "latest and greatest" therapies. Employers need to provide comprehensive benefits to attract and retain talented employees, but want to control the costs of these benefits. Health plans aim to meet the needs of the customer, although ultimately it is the employer who is primarily paying the bills. Finally, providers are struggling to maintain profitability and increase utilization. The fact that almost nowhere in the healthcare system is the customer also the purchaser results in a system that is focused primarily on price. When purchasers are the same as the customer, as in most other industries, more attention is focused on quality and value, as opposed to just cost. Although the Clinton administration attempted to initiate comprehensive healthcare reform in the early 1990s, the effort collapsed. However, if healthcare costs continue to rise sharply and the economy continues to slow, at some point, fundamental changes will be unavoidable.

Many believe that the country will eventually move toward a model in which the government is the single payer and provides national health insurance. The likelihood or timeframe for this happening is impossible to predict. However, it is clear that the government is becoming an increasingly important payer, especially as baby boomers move into Medicare eligibility, and programs like the Children's Health Insurance Program are introduced to expand coverage of special populations. In 1997, the government was responsible for more than 45 percent of total healthcare spending, which was an increase from 40.5 percent in 1990 (Healthcast 2010, 1999). The expanding role of government in the United States runs counter to what is happening in other countries. Most nations are trying to increase the level of privatization of healthcare and reduce government involvement.

Should the financing system maintain its present structure of multiple payers, one possibility for improvement could be the emergence of defined health benefit plans. Under such a plan, employers would provide a defined contribution to an employee, who would then select his or her benefit package, independent of the employer. This kind of approach has already occurred in the area of employees' retirement benefits. The Internet will be an important catalyst for moving health benefits to a defined contribution model, as will continued rising healthcare costs and increasing regulations and legislation. A recent survey of senior executives at *Fortune* 1000 companies revealed that almost 45 percent of respondents were either very interested or extremely interested in the defined contribution concept (National Center for Policy Analysis).

However, only a few organizations are currently offering defined contributions plans and very few employers have switched to this alternative model. Highmark Blue Cross Blue Shield, for example, is marketing a plan that enables small- and mid-sized employers to contribute a defined dollar amount for each employee. Each employee then selects the type of coverage he or she prefers, choosing from a range of co-payment, preventive services and drug coverage options.

One potential benefit of a shift to defined contribution could be an increased awareness of, and appreciation for, prevention and wellness programs among consumers, given the consumer ultimately will be more responsible and accountable for the cost of care.

How healthcare providers are paid is another complex and confounding element in the present healthcare system. Capitation was widely viewed as a reimbursement model that could transform the industry. Capitation requires providers, either individually or in a group, to take on risk for a defined patient population. But despite its early promise, capitation has not had the impact that was originally anticipated. Critics have been quick to denigrate this reimbursement method, insisting that it creates "perverse" economic incentives for the withholding of care. Such criticisms undoubtedly have helped ignite consumer indignation and backlash toward managed care generally. At the same time, many providers have feared that consumers would pursue litigation if they suspected care was inappropriately withheld.

Providers also have been unwilling to accept the risk of capitation because they have not had the cost and utilization data required to effectively manage capitated contracts. For those that have accepted such agreements, the results have not always been favorable. In 1999, the median income for physicians who received a significant amount of their income from capitation was lower than that of physicians who did not. Some large specialty groups – for example, the Denver-based Paramount IPA – were even forced to file bankruptcy (See Figure 28).

Currently, two out of three hospital executives surveyed reported that no aspect of the care their organizations deliver is capitated (US Hospitals and the Future of Health Care, 2000). Approximately 90 percent of hospitals report discounted fee-for-service as still their primary reimbursement model, followed by per diems (US Hospitals and the Future of Health Care, 2000). Additionally, the Medical Group Management Association reported that only 58 percent of multi-specialty medical groups had capitated

Figure 28. Providers Report Lower Average Capitation Rates
Source: Adapted with permission from the 1999 Capitation Survey: National Health Information, LLC., copyright 1999.

Average per-member, per-month rate:

	1997	1998	1999
All primary care services – Commercial	$11.98	$12.22	$11.07
All primary care services – Medicare	$22.27	$24.69	$28.87
All hospital services – Commercial	$40.70	$38.06	$35.76
All hospital services – Medicare	N/A	$156.95	$177.60

Figure 29. Capitation Declining in Provider Contracts
Source: Evergreen Re Inc., 1999

	1998	1999	Difference
Primary care	82%	83%	1%
Specialty physician	68%	59%	-9%
Hospital, inpatient	61%	50%	-11%
Hospital, outpatient	61%	50%	-11%
Emergency room	52%	41%	-11%
In-network only	48%	42%	-6%
Home health	47%	33%	-14%
Neonatal level II or III	40%	32%	-8%
Ambulance	40%	27%	-13%
Hospital, outpatient pharmaceuticals	34%	28%	-6%
Out-of-area services	34%	29%	-5%
Retail prescription pharmaceuticals	31%	25%	-6%
Transplants	28%	28%	0%

contracts, which are down from 68 percent in 1996, and capitated revenues accounted for only 11 percent of such groups' total revenues (See Figure 29). If capitation has any hope of becoming a viable reimbursement model, health plans must be willing to collaborate with capitated physicians to help them reduce risk and better manage patient populations. Plans could act as information intermediaries and share their utilization data to help all parties involved better manage care.

Strategic Implications for Healthcare Organizations

1. Understand the true costs of providing care and have internal experts capable of effectively and aggressively negotiating agreements with payers that allow for reasonable profit margins.

2. Assuming the emergence of a marketplace dominated by defined contribution plans, providers must increase marketing efforts to consumers to win their healthcare business. Creating a brand that is easily identifiable by consumers is an important first step in this process.

3. Again, assuming the increased prevalence of defined benefit plans, providers should consider developing a greater array of wellness and prevention services.

4. Disease management, utilization management and provider profiling techniques will be readily adopted by the industry and will be key attributes of future financing models.

Strategic Implications for Health Information Technology Organizations

1. Vendors need to create systems that are flexible and provide ongoing support for upgrades to avoid early system obsolescence in a rapidly changing reimbursement environment.

2. Special applications for utilization management will need to integrate with the primary clinical information systems of providers and other partners. Systems will also need to be customizable to adapt to unique provider pathways.

5.4 Competition for Capital

Background

More than many businesses, healthcare organizations continuously struggle to meet their business imperatives with limited resources. This is particularly true when it comes to access to capital. As a result, provider organizations are often forced to make difficult decisions about how to most effectively utilize their limited capital resources, whether it be to upgrade or build facilities, purchase equipment or maintain general operations.

Spending for information systems is another capital-intensive area, and, for a variety of reasons, healthcare investments in this area have lagged far behind those in other industries. Healthcare providers apparently are not yet convinced that information technology spending is worth sacrificing other priorities. An average health system spends 2.6 percent of its operating budget on information technology, although this figures varies with the size and complexity of information systems in an organization (Modern Healthcare, April 10, 2000, John's presentation). A Deloitte & Touche survey indicated that the majority of small hospitals anticipate spending up to $500,000 on information technology in the next year, while 32 percent of large hospitals projected that they would spend $5 million or more (US Hospitals and the Future of Health Care, 2000) (See Figure 30). In addition, spending on information technology has declined over the past two years, although most healthcare executives expect spending to increase in the next few years (US Hospitals and the Future of Health Care, 2000).

The healthcare organizations that are successful in acquiring capital will be those who have the data and information to convince investors of the organization's fundamental economic strength. Strong leadership also is important. Increasingly, many healthcare organizations have looked to the bond and stock market for capital. The number of initial public offerings and publicly traded healthcare organizations increased dramatically in the early to mid-1990s, although that growth has stabilized in the last few years. In fact, investment bankers and bond insurers have been decreasing their investments in healthcare and, as mentioned before, bond ratings for many not-for-profits have been downgraded, thereby increasing the cost of capital.

Figure 30. Healthcare Organizations Use of Charitable Gifts
Source: Modern Healthcare, July 31, 2000.

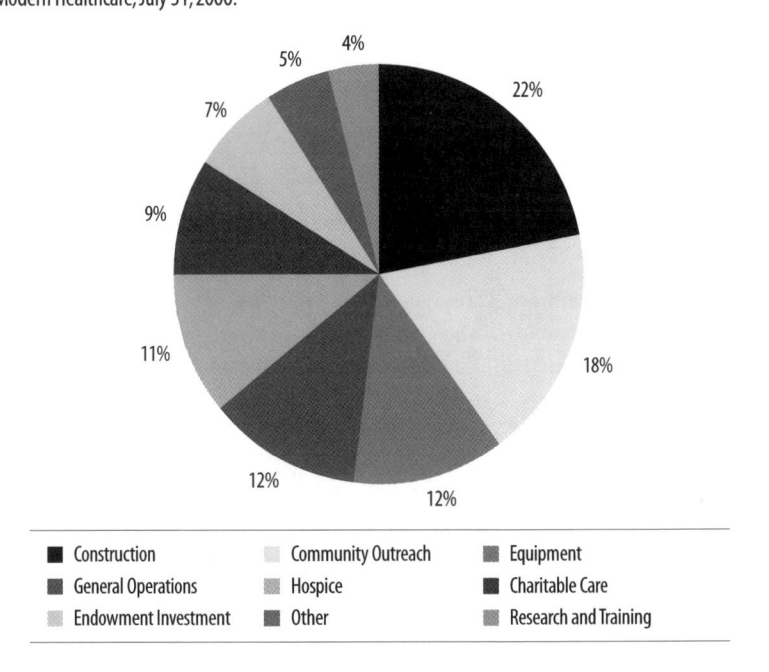

- Construction — 22%
- Community Outreach — 4%
- Equipment — 5%
- General Operations — 7%
- Hospice — 9%
- Charitable Care — 11%
- Endowment Investment — 12%
- Other — 12%
- Research and Training — 18%

Philanthropic organizations that support the delivery of healthcare have become popular sources for capital. Many healthcare organizations create foundations directly connected to their facilities. These organizations help raise funds for the clinical side of the operation, often from patients who had a positive experience with that facility or one of its providers. According to the Association for Healthcare Philanthropy, about $6 billion in charitable gifts were given to healthcare organizations in 1999 (Modern Healthcare, July 31, 2000). Charitable gifts are frequently used for large capital projects, such as those described in Figure 30. For example, the University of California Los Angeles Medical Center is relying on charitable gifts to cover the majority of their costs for a $1.2 billion capital project. Without these charitable contributions, healthcare organizations will be unable to grow, renovate or keep up with advances, especially in technology.

Strategic Implications for Healthcare Organizations
1. In the current financial environment, difficult cost-benefits decisions will continue to present themselves for provider organizations. Trade-offs between competing capital projects must be analyzed thoroughly to ensure the wisest use of limited resources. This analysis needs to take into account the manifold changes likely to occur in healthcare in the years ahead, as outlined in other sections of this document.
2. If consistent with organizational objectives, healthcare organizations should seek partnerships or joint ventures with entities that have the ability to contribute capital.

3. Foundations will continue to be an important source of funding. Strengthening these organizations and helping expand their fund-raising capabilities should be a high priority for non-profit entities.

Strategic Implications for Health Information Technology Organizations
1. HIT projects will continue to face intense competition for funding within healthcare organizations.
2. Vendors should create quantifiable, verifiable and replicable case studies that demonstrate the economic and clinical benefits of technology.
3. They should also examine all alternative financing mechanisms that may be available. These can include increasing the level of risk contracting whereby compensation is tied to performance metrics that enhance a provider's bottom line.
4. The speed to benefit realization should be enhanced. Much of the cynicism that surrounds provider perceptions of IT benefits arguably has been fueled by unrealistic representations about how quickly systems can produce a quantifiable ROI.
5. Vendors should consider offering an ASP-type financing model that effectively allows providers to lease IT systems on a pay-as-you-go basis. This would dramatically reduce up-front capital requirements for providers, while offering annuity-type revenue streams for vendors.

5.5 Costs of Healthcare Shift to Consumer

Background
Despite the rising costs of healthcare, consumers have, for the most part, been shielded from having to pay for the increases (See Figure 31). In fact, consumers' share of total health expenditures, which includes premium costs, co-payments and deductibles, fell from 34 percent in 1970 to 17 percent in 1999 (Healthcast 2010, 1999, p. 7). The transition to a managed care model contributed to decreased out-of-pocket outlays by consumers, since deductibles and co-payments are usually lower in managed care than in indemnity plans. However, that trend is beginning to reverse. Recent increases in premiums are leading employers to pass more of the costs on to individual employees. The number of medium and larger employers who are willing to cover the total cost of an employee's healthcare dropped from 64 percent in 1985 to 33 percent in 1995 (Center for Studying Health System Change, 1998). Additionally, the average co-payment for an HMO enrollee to visit the primary care physician rose from $4.36 in 1986 to $6.84 in 1996. Health plans also are designing benefits so that employees will be required to pay more for care. One example is the three-tier drug benefit formulary.

Figure 31. Average Monthly Employee Contribution for Single and Family Medical Coverage
Source: Bureau of Labor Statistics

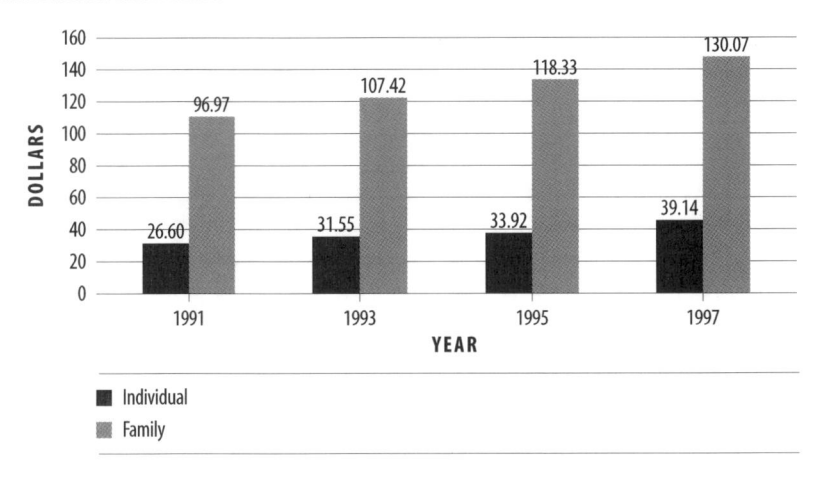

Year	Individual	Family
1991	26.60	96.97
1993	31.55	107.42
1995	33.92	118.33
1997	39.14	130.07

As the healthcare cost to consumers increases, they will begin to care more about utilization and value, especially if there is a trade-off between the two. Utilization could drop if consumers are unwilling or unable to cover their share of the cost. This phenomenon has already been seen with seniors who are unable to pay for their prescription drugs. Value will be a function of cost, quality, access and satisfaction.

Strategic Implications for Healthcare Organizations
1. Healthcare organizations must develop payment mechanisms that encourage consumers to be conscious of costs.
2. Providers should incorporate the concept of value into marketing efforts and, at some point, specifically craft messages targeting those individuals who are increasingly responsible for the cost of their care.
3. Providers must determine and actively market dimensions of value outside of cost.

Strategic Implications for Health Information Technology Organizations
1. HIT that can truly reduce costs will be implemented.
2. Vendors should market to consumers to let them know how HIT could reduce their cost of care, as well as provide a way to differentiate one provider from the next.
3. HIT could create convenience for the consumer, which would be worth the cost.

5.6 Integration/Consolidation

Background
In the decade between 1987 and 1997, more than 2,900 mergers and acquisitions occurred among healthcare organizations, including both providers and payers (See Figure 32). At the end of that period, the ten largest healthcare payers represented almost two-thirds of the total number of nationwide enrollees. Despite equally frenzied activity on the provider side, the top-ten hospital systems accounted for only 16 percent

Figure 32. Number of Health Care Mergers and Acquisitions
Source: Irving Levin Associates Inc.

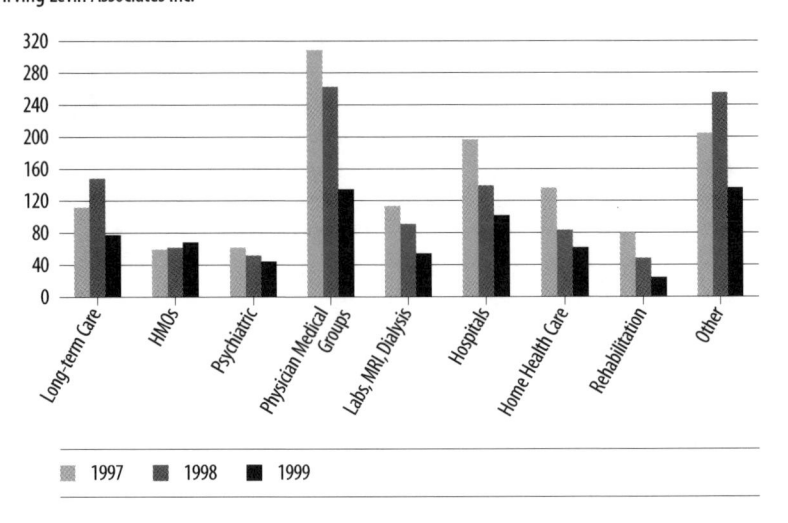

of the total inpatient beds in the country (Kaiser Family Foundation, 1998, p. 55). Since 1997, consolidation activity has declined, largely because of the lack of resources necessary to finance such activities, as well as the fact that the majority of healthcare collaborations have failed to meet expectations. In 2000, a total of 481 consolidation deals in all healthcare sectors were announced, a 34 percent decline from the previous year (Modern Healthcare, April 2, 2001).

For most healthcare organizations, the objectives of consolidation were to gain cost and operating efficiencies and market power. In theory, consolidated entities should have better access to patients, technology and capital, as well as the ability to leverage their size in contract negotiations. In reality, only one in three merged organizations were able to realize their objectives post-merger (US Hospitals and the Future of Health Care, 2000, p. 12). Some of the primary reasons for failure included the inability to merge services and cultures; lack of support from the physician community; failure to expand revenues; different missions (especially in terms of academic versus community hospitals, for-profit versus not-for-profit and religious versus secular); the cost of merging incompatible information systems; as well as the failure to consider the impact of public opinion.

Health plans that consolidated also hoped to benefit from cost efficiencies and market power, as well as decreased competition. They expected that lower levels of competition would allow them to charge higher rates. However, they soon discovered that buying market share did not always result in a profitable business.

When integration is achieved, it is often centered on administrative activities such as cost accounting and billing. In some cases, consolidated entities have been able to align and coordinate clinical services, such as lab, ambulatory care and emergency services (See Figure 33). However, only a few integrated systems have been able to merge their information systems (See Figure 34).

Figure 33. Levels of Integration: Systems Rate Their Efforts
Source: Shortell SM, et al. 2000. "Remaking Health Care in America: The Evolution of Organized Delivery Systems," 2nd ed. Jossey-Bass, San Francisco.

Integration Strategy	Average	Range
Meet population health needs	3.4	3.0 – 4.2
Match service capacity to population's needs	3.7	3.0 – 4.5
Integrate care across the continuum	3.5	3.0 – 4.0
Information systems link across the continuum	2.6	2.3 – 3.5
Provide info on costs and quality across system	3.8	3.0 – 4.5
Use financial incentives to align MDs and system	3.7	3.0 – 4.5
Continuously improve care	3.3	2.0 – 4.7
Work with others on community health needs	3.8	3.5 – 5.0

(Based on a Likert Scale of 1–5.)

Figure 34. Patient Care Services Combined or Eliminated When Part of a Larger Organization
Source: US Hospitals and the Future of Healthcare, page 14

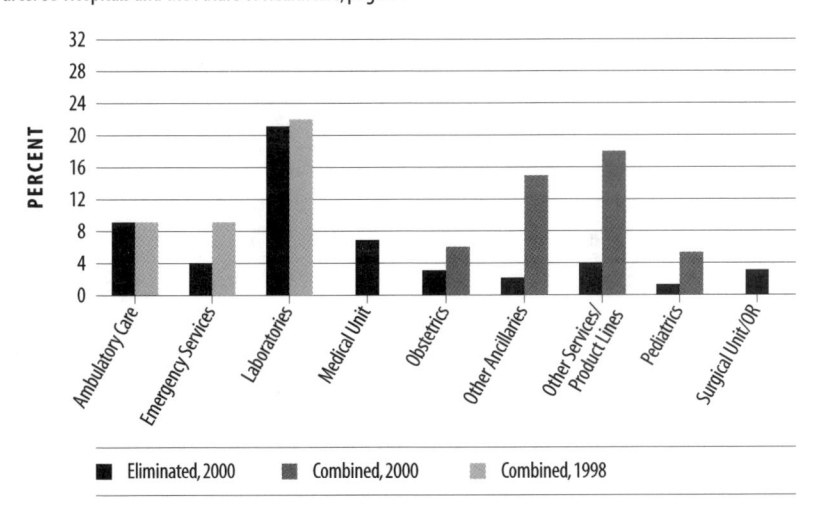

In general, mergers within one market and horizontal integration appear to be more successful than mergers across markets and vertical integration. When failures have occurred, as was the case for organizations like Penn State Geisinger Health System in Pennsylvania and UCSF-Stanford Health System in California, systems have chosen to disintegrate, returning organizations to their smaller, more manageable entities. Some of the most common disintegrations have involved hospitals or health systems divesting themselves of non-core businesses, such as health plans, physician groups or home healthcare companies (See Figure 35). Unfortunately, dissolving the consolidated entity can be more complicated than forming it in the first place.

Despite all of the merger and acquisition horror stories, consolidations will continue to play a role in the healthcare market. For example, Triad Hospitals plan to acquire Quorum Health Group this year, creating the third largest investor-owned hospital

Figure 35. System Components Health Systems Have Dropped
Source: Arista Associates, 1999

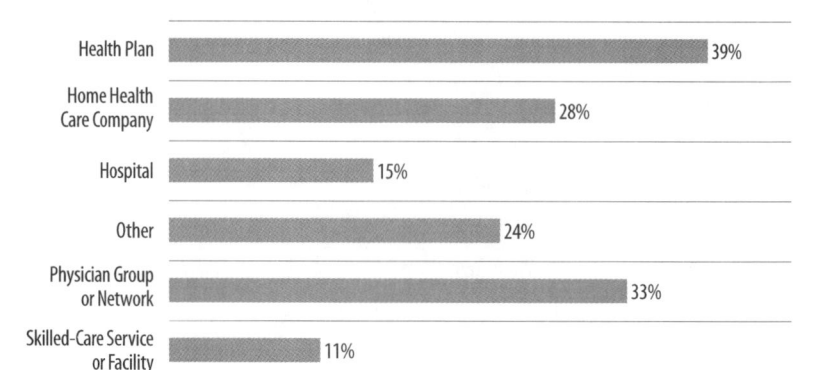

Component	Percentage
Health Plan	39%
Home Health Care Company	28%
Hospital	15%
Other	24%
Physician Group or Network	33%
Skilled-Care Service or Facility	11%

corporation. The combined entity will own 53 hospitals. HCA-The Healthcare Co. and Tenet, two large for-profit hospital systems, are also likely to continue to seek strategic acquisitions. Rural community hospitals in need of capital are prime targets for acquisition. For those organizations who continue to consider consolidation as a viable strategy, their ability to complete proper due diligence will contribute to their success and help them avoid the path of failure that has been paved by so many other healthcare organizations.

Strategic Implications for Healthcare Organizations

1. Providers should be clear about expectations of consolidation from the outset. At the same time, the objectives of a merger should be clearly enumerated for all constituencies, including employees, customers and vendors.

2. Despite hopes that mergers and acquisitions would successfully mesh previously disparate healthcare entities into consolidated organizations with broad, efficient and market dominant scopes of services, few success stories have emerged. Relative to mergers and acquisitions, healthcare organizations should proceed with caution, assessing organizational cultures and philosophies of care, business plans and strategies, care delivery models and information systems.

3. As the cost of healthcare shifts more to consumers (See Section 5.5), value, especially those dimensions of value associated with quality (e.g., clinical excellence, ease of access, convenience, timeliness of service delivery, satisfaction, etc.) will become of paramount importance to healthcare organizations attempting to gain competitive differentiation. Fully integrated organizations that offer convenient access to a wide variety of cost-effective services in a variety of locations will be ideally positioned within virtually any marketplace to deliver value-driven healthcare.

Strategic Implications for Health Information Technology Organizations
1. Mergers and acquisitions will continue to create opportunities for HIT organizations as providers struggle to interface existing IT systems or purchase and implement new IT systems.

2. As healthcare organizations seek to expand the administrative benefits realized through consolidation into the clinical realm, a wide array of opportunities will emerge around clinical data systems alignment.

3. The broader sharing of patient data across a consolidated enterprise will mandate greater security measures to ensure HIPAA compliance.

4. As healthcare organizations consolidate physically and operationally, they will also need to consolidate virtually in terms of availability of patient information across a variety of care delivery locations. Opportunities will emerge for HIT vendors who are able to facilitate this virtual consolidation.

Section 6.0 – Health Policy

6.1 Medicare and Medicaid Reform

Background

Recent reports indicate that the Medicare Hospital Insurance Trust Fund, which covers the costs of hospital, nursing home and other institutional care for Medicare beneficiaries, is now expected to remain solvent through 2029 – an improvement from a 1998 projection that predicted solvency only through 2009. This revised forecast has been attributed to the Balanced Budget Act of 1997, efforts to reduce fraud and abuse, and slower than expected growth in healthcare costs and Medicare spending. However, the long-term stability of the fund and the entire Medicare program remains threatened, especially if attempts to enrich the benefits provided to Medicare beneficiaries without identifying additional funding sources succeed. Additionally, Medicare spending continues to rise (See Figure 36). As a result, efforts to implement Medicare and Medicaid reform ensue.

Transitioning some of the Medicare and Medicaid enrollees into health maintenance organizations has been one approach taken to revitalize and privatize the Medicare and Medicaid programs. While the enrollment in these special HMOs has been growing, many of the private health plans that offer these products have recently withdrawn from the programs or from specific service areas as a result of inadequate reimbursement. In response to the withdrawals, Congress increased reimbursement to Medicare HMOs by an average of 5.3 percent in most service areas with the passage of the Benefits Improvement and Protection Act (BIPA) in December 1999. As a result, a few plans have chosen to reenter certain markets, but their long-term commitment to the program is questionable

A second strategy to control Medicare spending is the introduction of an outpatient prospective payment system (OPPS), which is similar to the DRG methodology that is used to cover the cost of inpatient care for Medicare beneficiaries. Implemented in

Figure 36. Medicare Spending
Source: Health Care Financing Administration

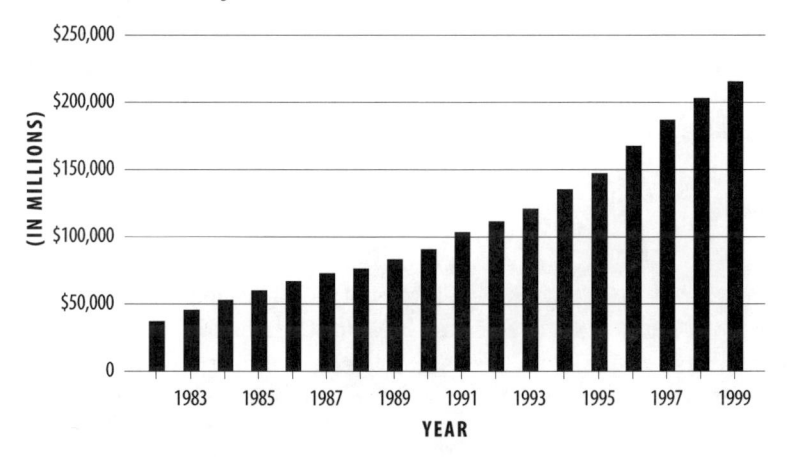

August 2000, OPPS provides acute and psychiatric hospital-based outpatient facilities with a fixed dollar amount for services based on ambulatory payment classifications (APCs). This payment method is thought to encourage providers to manage resource usage efficiently. The change in reimbursement methodology is projected to save the Medicare program more than $6 billion in the next three years, with hospitals receiving on average 3.8 percent less reimbursement for outpatient services.

Another area of possible reform is the addition of a pharmacy benefit to Medicare. Although this change would increase Medicare costs, it is viewed as a significant shortcoming in the current system and many seniors want the issue addressed. Only about one-third of individuals over the age of 65 currently have adequate prescription drug coverage (Center for Studying Health System Change, 2000). Although the prescription drug benefit was an important platform for the 2000 presidential election, it is still uncertain what the ultimate outcome of this issue will be. What is known is that with drug costs rising, there may not be enough money in the federal 2001-2002 budget to add a benefit. Consequently, the issue is likely to continue to be debated this year.

As more of the population approaches the age at which they will qualify for Medicare benefits, the emphasis on reform will become more important to politicians and therefore the likelihood for change will increase. And because the government is such a large payer, any changes to Medicare or Medicaid will dramatically affect the entire healthcare system.

Strategic Implications for Healthcare Organizations
1. The Medicare population can be expected to increase as the baby-boomer generation ages. At the same time, provider reimbursements can be expected to decrease as the outpatient payment system is phased in. These trends will lead to an overall decrease in revenue for provider organizations.

2. If the proposed Medicare drug benefits are passed, the benefit structure of health plans offering either supplemental or managed care coverage to Medicare recipients must be redefined.

Strategic Implications for Health Information Technology Organizations
Diminished Medicare reimbursements will place added pressure on provider organizations to maximize the efficiency and effectiveness of their care delivery processes. HIT vendors who have quantifiable and reproducible evidence of their systems' ability to help create "smoothly operating factories of care" that produce efficient and effective outcomes will be rewarded by the market place.

6.2 The Uninsured

Background
In 1998, almost 45 million Americans, or 18 percent of the population, was uninsured – a 43 percent increase from 1987 (See Figure 37). However, in 1999, the number of uninsured dropped by about 1.7 million, largely as a result of increased employment levels and the strong economy. Although it is hoped that this trend will continue, it

Figure 37. Number of Uninsured Americans
Source: US Census Bureau, 4700 Silver Hill Road, Suitland, MD 20743, www.census.gov

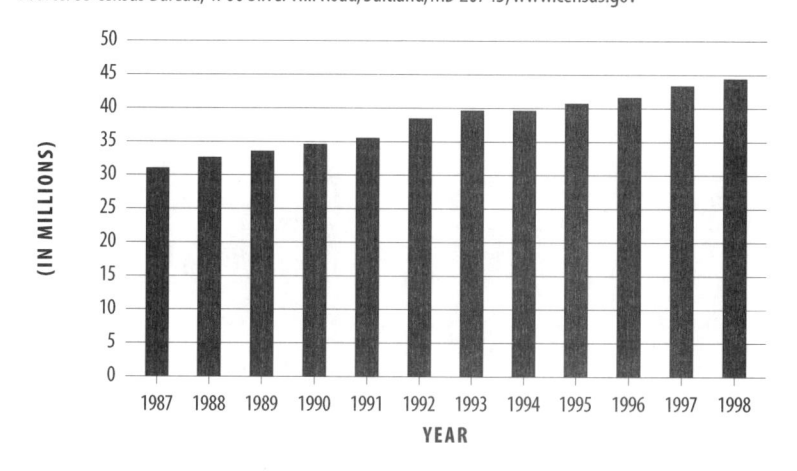

will likely take more than economic improvements to eliminate the number of people not covered by health insurance, especially since a majority of the uninsured population are the working poor – individuals who have jobs but who make too much money to qualify for Medicaid and too little to purchase private or employer-sponsored coverage. Many of the working poor are young people; more than 30 percent of individuals between the ages of 18 and 24 are uninsured. Approximately 15 percent of the uninsured are children, but thanks to the Children's Health Insurance Program, this number has been decreasing. Additionally, racial and ethnic differences are evident in the composition of the uninsured population. For example, Hispanics are three times more likely to be uninsured than non-Hispanic whites.

The American Hospital Association estimates that an average of 6 percent of a hospital's budget is spent on uncompensated care (See Figure 38). Not-for-profit hospitals and public health departments provide greater than their share of care for the uninsured. The burden of providing charity care is growing, especially since providers can no longer subsidize this care through higher reimbursement from other payers. In some cases, the financial burden has caused hospitals to close their doors. For example, D.C. General Hospital, a public institution in the District of Columbia that was founded in the early 1800s, will close later this year because the government is no longer able to provide funds for it to continue operations. In 1996, D.C. General provided more than $75 million in uncompensated care. The impact of closing facilities like D.C. General could create geographic gaps in coverage and could negatively impact the bottom line of numerous facilities that become the recipients of increased uninsured patient loads.

To date, no comprehensive plans to address the issue of the uninsured have been formulated, although several pieces of legislation have been drafted to present to Congress this year. Solutions include expanding state level programs like the Children's Health Insurance Program (CHIP), providing incentives for employers to offer coverage, creating tax credits for workers who purchase healthcare coverage,

Figure 38. Hospitals' Uncompensated-care Costs
Source: Hospital Statistics

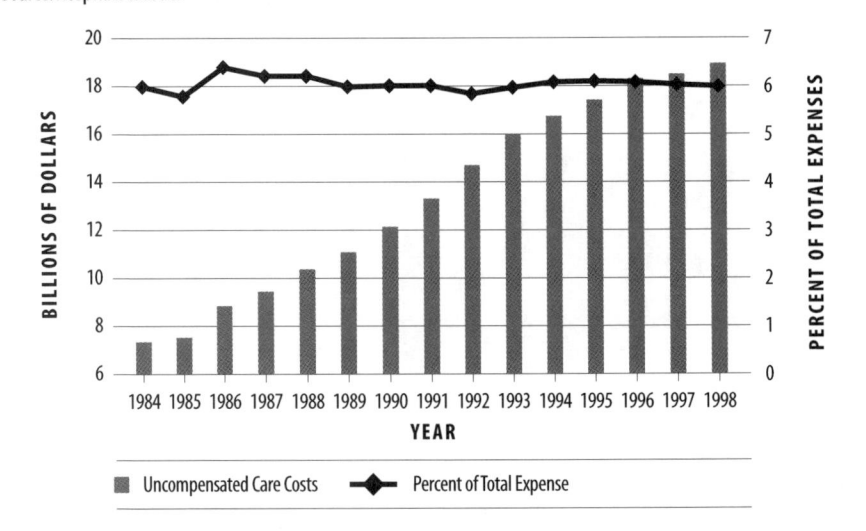

allowing health insurance premiums to be tax deductible and encouraging the use of medical savings accounts. Despite the public interest in the problem of the uninsured, most insured Americans believe it is the government's responsibility to address the problem. They believe that they neither can nor should play an active role in helping to solve this national crisis.

Strategic Implications for Healthcare Organizations
The expanding number of uninsured represents a major concern for healthcare organizations, especially not-for-profit entities. Healthcare organizations must actively support legislation to expand coverage to the broadest range of individuals possible.

Strategic Implications for Health Information Technology Organizations
HIT organizations must recognize that the large number of uninsured represents a significant economic burden to healthcare organizations – particularly major academic medical centers. As such, the HIT community should be proactive in both exploring innovative solutions to this perplexing problem, as well as adding its voice to the providers' lobbying efforts.

Section 7.0 – Human Capital

7.1 Human Resource Shortages

Background

Healthcare is necessarily human resources-intensive. When qualified staff are not available, services cannot be delivered. Therefore, maintaining adequate staffing levels is critical for healthcare organizations. However, this will become increasingly difficult in the future.

For a range of reasons, including inadequate pay, difficult physical conditions, and an expanding array of employment opportunities for women outside of healthcare, the nursing profession will be among the hardest hit areas in terms of shortages. The average age of a nurse currently is 44 years, and new nurses are not entering the field fast enough to replace those who are retiring (Futurescan, 2001). Enrollment in bachelor's-degree nursing programs has fallen over the last five years, tumbling 4.6 percent in 1999 alone. Even masters' level programs, which had seen steady enrollment growth in the 1990s, are experiencing enrollment declines. The inability of most healthcare organizations to offer the competitive compensation packages, when compared to other sectors, along with increasingly difficult working conditions, has seriously eroded the profession's allure. Almost 55 percent of nurses who responded to a survey by the American Nursing Association indicated that they would not recommend their profession to friends or their children. Acute care nursing has developed a reputation for being a high-stress, under-appreciated and often physically demanding profession. As a result, many qualified nurses are applying their experience in the array of new opportunities outside of patient care, including in managed care positions and in pharmaceutical research and sales.

Pharmacists, physical therapists, radiation technologists and other ancillary service providers, such as information technologists, also will be in short supply in the years ahead. The Pharmacy Manpower Project, a consortium of pharmacists and pharmaceutical associations, estimates that the nationwide demand for pharmacists is 4.1 on a scale of 1 to 5 (Hospitals and Health Networks, October 2000). Like nurses, pharmacists have a wide range of opportunities outside the acute care setting, most notably in the retail sector, where chain store growth is fueling higher salaries. Jobs in fields like information technology will be especially hard to fill because the demand is driven by all industries, not just healthcare. Recruiting these individuals will be very competitive and may require special tactics.

Although physicians, in general, are not in short supply, there are some specialties in which demand exceeds supply. For example, intensivists and hospitalists are in heavy demand. Payers and business coalitions have encouraged the use of these super-specialists, and doctors and consumers have begun to realize their benefit. Hospitalists have been shown to help reduce inpatient stays by more than 20 percent and help cut hospital costs by 20 percent (Futurescan, 2001 from Chesanow, 1998). The shortage among specialists, including radiologists, was to a large extent set in motion by the

Figure 39. Response to Staff Shortages
Source: US Hospitals and the Future of Healthcare, page 46.

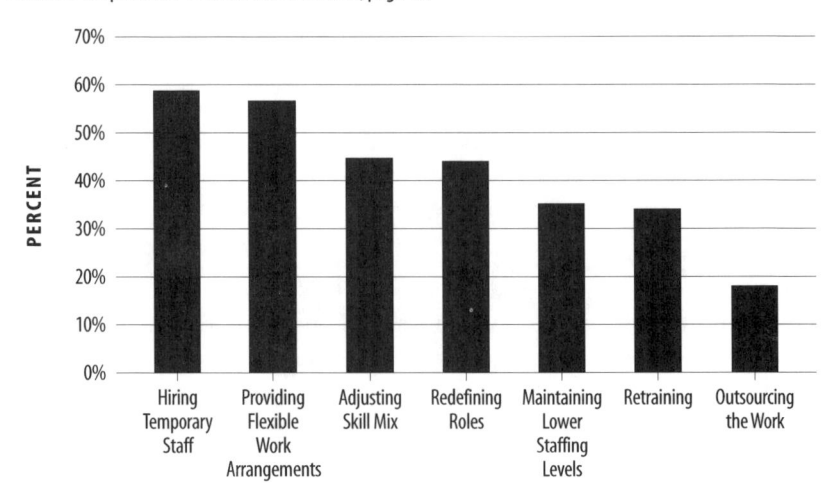

Response	Percent
Hiring Temporary Staff	~59%
Providing Flexible Work Arrangements	~57%
Adjusting Skill Mix	~45%
Redefining Roles	~44%
Maintaining Lower Staffing Levels	~35%
Retraining	~34%
Outsourcing the Work	~18%

erroneous assumptions regarding the declining role of specialists made in the healthcare reform tumult of the early to -mid-1990s.

To prevent the disruption of service going forward, healthcare organizations already are implementing special recruitment and retention strategies for select positions. Some of the most common enticements include offering signing bonuses, high salaries, relocation reimbursement and other incentive packages (See Figure 39). Some facilities are also outsourcing activities, when possible, and utilizing temporary staffing. Although all of these strategies could potentially lessen the impact of shortages, the most successful organizations are likely to be those that acknowledge the importance of employee satisfaction and actively work to retain existing staff by empowering them with substantive roles in organizational decision-making.

Strategic Implications for Healthcare Organizations

1. Declining nursing program enrollments means that the current nursing shortage will not be alleviated by new influxes of graduating nurses. Consequently, retention becomes critical for organizations wishing to avoid service interruptions.

2. Although higher wages and incentives are important components in retention strategies, surveys show that the physically challenging working conditions and perceived lack of status or respect within healthcare organizations are major reasons for the flight from the nursing profession. Providers therefore must make cultural changes that explicitly and implicitly recognize and reward the role nurses play at the core of the acute care experience. The traditional perception among many administrators that nurses are simply another interchangeable labor commodity is archaic and self-defeating.

3. On a wider front, healthcare organizations must develop programs that emphasize the rewards of a healthcare profession to students at earlier ages to boost enrollment in the healthcare educational pipeline.

4. Organizations must also lobby for changes in immigration laws, which would allow trained nurses from countries where nursing surpluses exist to work in the United States.

5. Outsourcing will become increasingly important in areas like food service and laundry because of the inability to hire entry-level personnel.

6. Tools that can reduce the administrative burden on front-line healthcare workers – notably information automation systems – are critical selling points in the recruitment and retention of clinical staff.

Strategic Implications for Health Information Technology Organizations

1. An emphasis on the labor-saving aspects of information technologies will be an increasingly important selling point for IT vendors.

2. The continued refinement in time-saving technologies, including voice recognition systems, will give technology companies an advantage as providers scramble to adapt to chronic labor shortages.

7.2 Unionization

Background

Healthcare has traditionally been a non-unionized industry, although the number of healthcare employees represented by unions has been growing. A 1994 Modern Healthcare survey reported that 25 percent of U.S. hospitals have at least one collective bargaining union represented within their facility. The Service Employees International Union represents the largest number of healthcare workers, with members ranging from hospital housekeeping staff to a small number of physicians and nurses. The unionization of physicians and nurses has been a recent phenomenon and, to date, only 6 percent of the nation's 757,000 physicians and 17 percent of the 2.6 million nurses are unionized. Up until last year, the American Medical Association (AMA) opposed physicians joining unions. Now, however, the AMA is forming its own collective negotiating unit for employed physicians, and the organization should be operational by the summer of 2001.

The recent rise of unionization has been largely attributed to what has been described as an increasingly hostile healthcare environment. Healthcare employees report long hours, inadequate reimbursement, delayed payments from managed care organizations, concerns about the quality of care, inappropriate staffing ratios and the loss of autonomy as primary reasons for considering unionization. Employees see unions as a way to find a collective voice that can resist some of these poor conditions.

Administrators of healthcare organizations view unions as third-party organizations that make negotiating directly with employees more difficult. As a result, they are working to meet employees' needs so that unionization sentiment does not grow. Whether or not they will be successful and to what extent unionization will take firm root in the healthcare industry remains to be seen.

Strategic Implications for Healthcare Organizations
1. Demonstrating an understanding of the conditions many healthcare workers labor under and working to improve those conditions is an important strategy for diminishing the allure of unions. Similarly, simply maintaining open and effective communications between administrators and line workers can pay major dividends in terms of avoiding staff alienation.

2. Maintaining good relationships with unions if and when they do form will help avoid the kind of worker rancor and ill will that can trigger a diminution in the quality of care.

Strategic Implications for Health Information Technology Organizations
HIT vendors may choose to work with unions to advocate for the adoption of technologies to ease the pressures on healthcare workers and reduce medical errors.